Update in Hospital Medicine

Editor

ANDREW S. DUNN

MEDICAL CLINICS OF NORTH AMERICA

www.medical.theclinics.com

Consulting Editor
JACK ENDE

July 2020 • Volume 104 • Number 4

ELSEVIER

1600 John F. Kennedy Boulevard ⚫ Suite 1800 ⚫ Philadelphia, Pennsylvania, 19103-2899

http://www.theclinics.com

MEDICAL CLINICS OF NORTH AMERICA Volume 104, Number 4
July 2020 ISSN 0025-7125, ISBN-13: 978-0-323-75722-5

Editor: Katerina Heidhausen
Developmental Editor: Kristen Helm

Medical Clinics of North America (ISSN 0025-7125) is published bimonthly by Elsevier Inc., 360 Park Avenue South, New York, NY 10010-1710. Months of publication are January, March, May, July, September, and November. Business and editorial offices: 1600 John F. Kennedy Boulevard, Suite 1800, Philadelphia, PA 19103-2899. Periodicals postage paid at New York, NY, and additional mailing offices. Subscription prices are USD $295.00 per year (US individuals), $654.00 per year (US institutions), $100.00 per year (US Students), $353.00 per year (Canadian individuals), $850.00 per year (Canadian institutions), $200.00 per year for (foreign students), $100.00 per year for (Canadian students), $422.00 per year (foreign individuals), and $850.00 per year (foreign institutions). To receive student/resident rate, orders must be accompanied by name of affiliated institution, date of term, and the signature of program/residency coordinator on institution letterhead. Orders will be billed at individual rate until proof of status is received. Foreign air speed delivery is included in all Clinics' subscription prices. All prices are subject to change without notice. **POSTMASTER:** Send address changes to *Medical Clinics of North America*, Elsevier Health Sciences Division, Subscription Customer Service, 3251 Riverport Lane, Maryland Heights, MO 63043. **Customer Service: Telephone: 1-800-654-2452** (U.S. and Canada); **1-314-447-8871** (outside U.S. and Canada). **Fax: 314-447-8029. E-mail: journalscustomerserviceusa@elsevier.com** (for print support); **journalsonlinesupport-usa@elsevier.com** (for online support).

Reprints. For copies of 100 or more of articles in this publication, please contact the Commercial Reprints Department, Elsevier Inc., 360 Park Avenue South, New York, NY 10010-1710. Tel.: 212-633-3874; Fax: 212-633-3820; E-mail: reprints@elsevier.com.

Medical Clinics of North America is also published in Spanish by McGraw-Hill Interamericana Editores S. A., P.O. Box 5-237, 06500 Mexico, D.F., Mexico.

Medical Clinics of North America is covered in *MEDLINE/PubMed (Index Medicus), Current Contents, ASCA, Excerpta Medica, Science Citation Index,* and *ISI/BIOMED.*

PROGRAM OBJECTIVE

The goal of the *Medical Clinics of North America* is to keep practicing physicians up to date with current clinical practice by providing timely articles reviewing the state of the art in patient care.

TARGET AUDIENCE

All practicing physicians and other healthcare professionals.

LEARNING OBJECTIVES

Upon completion of this activity, participants will be able to:

1. Review hospitalists medicine group plan to improve performance and teamwork based on retention, development, and a commitment to communication.
2. Explain common manifestations and treatment options of excessive alcohol intake and opioid use disorder.
3. Discuss diagnosis and treatment using evidence-based recommendations for sepsis/septic shock, congestive heart failure, venous thromboembolism, pneumonia, acute liver injury and catheter-associated urinary tract infections.

ACCREDITATION

The Elsevier Office of Continuing Medical Education (EOCME) is accredited by the Accreditation Council for Continuing Medical Education (ACCME) to provide continuing medical education for physicians.

The EOCME designates this journal-based CME activity for a maximum of 12 *AMA PRA Category 1 Credit*(s)™. Physicians should claim only the credit commensurate with the extent of their participation in the activity.

All other healthcare professionals requesting continuing education credit for this enduring material will be issued a certificate of participation.

DISCLOSURE OF CONFLICTS OF INTEREST

The EOCME assesses conflict of interest with its instructors, faculty, planners, and other individuals who are in a position to control the content of CME activities. All relevant conflicts of interest that are identified are thoroughly vetted by EOCME for fair balance, scientific objectivity, and patient care recommendations. EOCME is committed to providing its learners with CME activities that promote improvements or quality in healthcare and not a specific proprietary business or a commercial interest.

The planning committee, staff, authors and editors listed below have identified no financial relationships or relationships to products or devices they or their spouse/life partner have with commercial interest related to the content of this CME activity:

Jesse Abelson, MD; Stacey-Ann Whittaker Brown, MD, MPH; Abigail Bryne, MD; Svetlana Chernyavsky, DO; Vineet Chopra, MD, MSc; James F. Crismale, MD; Rachel M. Cyrus, MD; Patricia Dharapak, MD; Jack Ende, MD, MACP; Matthew Fine; Michael D. Font, MD; Scott L. Friedman, MD; Nina Garza, DO, MPH; Matt George, MD; Krystal Hanrahan, MS, MSPH, RN, CMSRN; Kristen Helm; Michael Herscher, MD, MA; Leeza Hirt; Jennifer Hui, MD; Abraham Kanal, MD; Eric Kaplovitch, MD; Marilu Kelly, MSN, RN, CNE, CHCP; Ashish K. Khanna, MD, FCCP, FCCM; Violetta Laskova, MD; Matthew Luzum, MD, MPH; Eve Merrill, MD; Sashi Nair, MD; Reema Navalurkar; Kevin J. O'Leary, MD, MS; Kamana Pillay, MD; Dahlia Rizk, DO, MPH; Jonathan Sebolt, MD; Bradley A. Sharpe, MD; Joseph R. Shaw, MD; Evan Siau, MD; Jeyanthi Surendrakumar; Braghadheeswar Thyagarajan, MD; Linda Wang, MD; Jeff Wiese, MD.

The planning committee, staff, authors and editors listed below have identified financial relationships or relationships to products or devices they or their spouse/life partner have with commercial interest related to the content of this CME activity:

Sidney Braman, MD, Master FCCP: consultant/advisor for AstraZeneca; speaker's bureau for Genentech, Inc. James Douketis, MD, FRCP: personal fees from Janssen Pharmaceuticals, Inc., Pfizer Inc, Bayer AG, Bristol Myers Squibb Company, Sanofi-Aventis U.S. LLC, Servier, and Portola Pharmaceuticals, Inc. Andrew S. Dunn, MD, MPH, SFHM, MACP: research support from Pfizer Inc.; consultant/advisor for Bristol Myers Squibb Company, Scott Kaatz, DO, MSc: consultant for Bristol Myers Squibb Company, Pfizer Inc., Portola Pharmaceuticals, Inc., and F. Hoffmann-La Roche Ltd; consultant/advisor and research support from Janssen Pharmaceuticals, Inc. Sumeet Singh Mitter, MD, MSc: speaker's bureau for Abbott, Sean P. Pinney, MD: consultant/advisor for Abbott, CareDx, Medtronic, and Procyrion, Inc.

UNAPPROVED/OFF-LABEL USE DISCLOSURE

The EOCME requires CME faculty to disclose to the participants:

1. When products or procedures being discussed are off-label, unlabelled, experimental, and/or investigational (not US Food and Drug Administration [FDA] approved); and
2. Any limitations on the information presented, such as data that are preliminary or that represent ongoing research, interim analyses, and/or unsupported opinions. Faculty may discuss information about pharmaceutical agents that is outside of FDA-approved labelling. This information is intended solely for CME and is not intended to promote off-label use of these medications. If you have any questions, contact the medical affairs department of the manufacturer for the most recent prescribing information.

TO ENROLL

To enroll in the *Medical Clinics of North America* Continuing Medical Education program, call customer service at 1-800-654-2452 or sign up online at http://www.theclinics.com/home/cme. The CME program is available to subscribers for an additional annual fee of USD 300.00.

METHOD OF PARTICIPATION

In order to claim credit, participants must complete the following;

1. Complete enrolment as indicated above.
2. Read the activity.
3. Complete the CME Test and Evaluation. Participants must achieve a score of 70% on the test. All CME Tests and Evaluations must be completed online.

CME INQUIRIES/SPECIAL NEEDS

For all CME inquiries or special needs, please contact elsevierCME@elsevier.com.

MEDICAL CLINICS OF NORTH AMERICA

FORTHCOMING ISSUES

September 2020
Geriatrics
Danelle Cayea, *Editor*

November 2020
Cancer Prevention and Screening
Robert A. Smith and Kevin Oeffinger,
Editors

January 2021
Common Symptoms in Outpatient Practice
Lia S. Logio, *Editor*

RECENT ISSUES

May 2020
Palliative Care
Eric Widera, *Editor*

March 2020
**Physical Medicine and Rehabilitation: An
Update for Internists**
David A. Lenrow, *Editor*

January 2020
Allergy and Immunology for the Internist
Anne Marie Ditto *Editor*

SERIES OF RELATED INTEREST

Physician Assistant Clinics
https://www.physicianassistant.theclinics.com/
Primary Care: Clinics in Office Practice
https://www.primarycare.theclinics.com/

Contributors

CONSULTING EDITOR

JACK ENDE, MD, MACP
The Schaeffer Professor of Medicine, Perelman School of Medicine, University of Pennsylvania, Philadelphia, Pennsylvania, USA

EDITOR

ANDREW S. DUNN, MD, MPH, SFHM, MACP
Professor of Medicine, Chief, Division of Hospital Medicine, Mount Sinai Health System, New York, New York, USA

AUTHORS

JESSE ABELSON, MD
Assistant Clinical Professor, Division of Hospital Medicine, Department of Medicine, University of California, San Francisco (UCSF), San Francisco, California, USA

SIDNEY BRAMAN, MD, Master FCCP
Division of Pulmonary, Critical Care and Sleep Medicine, Icahn School of Medicine at Mount Sinai, New York, New York, USA

ABIGAIL BRYNE, MD
Department of Internal Medicine, Tulane University, New Orleans, Louisiana, USA

SVETLANA CHERNYAVSKY, DO
Hospitalist, Department of Medicine, Mount Sinai Beth Israel, Assistant Professor, Icahn School of Medicine at Mount Sinai, New York, New York, USA

VINEET CHOPRA, MD, MSc
Division of Hospital Medicine, Department of Medicine, University of Michigan, Ann Arbor, Michigan, USA

JAMES F. CRISMALE, MD
Assistant Professor, Division of Liver Diseases, Department of Medicine, Icahn School of Medicine at Mount Sinai, New York, New York, USA

RACHEL M. CYRUS, MD
Assistant Professor and Director of Clinical Operations, Division of Hospital Medicine, Northwestern University Feinberg School of Medicine, Chicago, Illinois, USA

PATRICIA DHARAPAK, MD
Hospitalist, Department of Medicine, Mount Sinai Beth Israel, Assistant Professor, Icahn School of Medicine at Mount Sinai, New York, New York, USA

JAMES DOUKETIS, MD, FRCP(C)
Department of Medicine, Divisions of General Internal Medicine, and Hematology and Thromboembolism, McMaster University, St. Joseph's Healthcare Hamilton, Hamilton, Canada

MATTHEW FINE
Department of Medical Education, Icahn School of Medicine at Mount Sinai, New York, New York, USA

MICHAEL D. FONT, MD
Resident, Department of Anesthesiology, Wake Forest School of Medicine, Wake Forest Baptist Medical Center, Winston-Salem, North Carolina, USA

SCOTT L. FRIEDMAN, MD
Dean for Therapeutic Discovery, Fishberg Professor of Medicine, Professor of Pharmacologic Sciences, Chief - Division of Liver Diseases, Department of Medicine, Icahn School of Medicine at Mount Sinai, New York, New York, USA

NINA GARZA, DO, MPH
Chief Medical Resident, Department of Medicine, Henry Ford Hospital, Detroit, Michigan, USA

MATT GEORGE, MD
Director of Observation Medicine, Division of Hospital Medicine, Henry Ford West Bloomfield Hospital, West Bloomfield, Michigan, USA

KRYSTAL HANRAHAN, MS, MSPH, RN, CMSRN
Nursing Development, Magnet Program Manager, Northwestern Memorial Hospital, Chicago, Illinois, USA

MICHAEL HERSCHER, MD, MA
Assistant Professor, Division of Hospital Medicine, Department of Medicine, Icahn School of Medicine at Mount Sinai, New York, New York, USA

LEEZA HIRT
Department of Medical Education, Icahn School of Medicine at Mount Sinai, New York, New York, USA

JENNIFER HUI, MD
Hospitalist, Department of Medicine, Mount Sinai Beth Israel, Assistant Professor, Icahn School of Medicine at Mount Sinai, New York, New York, USA

SCOTT KAATZ, DO, MSc
Medical Director for Professional Development and Research, Division of Hospital Medicine, Henry Ford Hospital, Clinical Professor of Medicine, Wayne State University, Detroit, Michigan, USA

ABRAHAM KANAL, MD
Assistant Clinical Professor, Division of Hospital Medicine, Department of Medicine, University of California, San Francisco (UCSF), San Francisco, California, USA

ERIC KAPLOVITCH, MD
Department of Medicine, University Health Network, University of Toronto, Toronto, Ontario, Canada

ASHISH K. KHANNA, MD, FCCP, FCCM
Associate Professor, Section Head for Research, Department of Anesthesiology, Section on Critical Care Medicine, Wake Forest School of Medicine, Wake Forest Baptist Medical Center, Winston-Salem, North Carolina, USA; Outcomes Research Consortium, Cleveland, Ohio, USA

VIOLETTA LASKOVA, MD
Hospitalist, Department of Medicine, Mount Sinai Beth Israel, Assistant Professor, Icahn School of Medicine at Mount Sinai, New York, New York, USA

MATTHEW LUZUM, MD, MPH
Division of Hospital Medicine, Department of Medicine, University of Michigan, Ann Arbor, Michigan, USA

EVE MERRILL, MD
Hospitalist, Department of Medicine, Mount Sinai Beth Israel, Assistant Professor, Icahn School of Medicine at Mount Sinai, New York, New York, USA

SUMEET S. MITTER, MD, MSc, FACC
Assistant Professor of Medicine, Icahn School of Medicine at Mount Sinai, New York, New York, USA

SASHI NAIR, MD
Medical Resident, Department of Medicine, Henry Ford Hospital, Detroit, Michigan, USA

REEMA NAVALURKAR
Department of Medical Education, Icahn School of Medicine at Mount Sinai, New York, New York, USA

KEVIN J. O'LEARY, MD, MS
Professor and Chief, Division of Hospital Medicine, Northwestern University Feinberg School of Medicine, Chicago, Illinois, USA

KAMANA PILLAY, MD
Hospitalist, Department of Medicine, Mount Sinai Beth Israel, Assistant Professor, Icahn School of Medicine at Mount Sinai, New York, New York, USA

SEAN P. PINNEY, MD, FACC
Professor of Medicine, Icahn School of Medicine at Mount Sinai, New York, New York, USA

DAHLIA RIZK, DO, MPH
Chief, Division of Hospital Medicine, Department of Medicine, Mount Sinai Beth Israel, Associate Professor, Icahn School of Medicine at Mount Sinai, New York, New York, USA

JONATHAN SEBOLT, MD
Division of Hospital Medicine, Department of Medicine, University of Michigan, Ann Arbor, Michigan, USA

BRADLEY A. SHARPE, MD
Professor of Clinical Medicine, Division of Hospital Medicine, Department of Medicine, University of California, San Francisco (UCSF), San Francisco, California, USA

JOSEPH R. SHAW, MD
Ottawa Blood Disease Center, Division of Hematology, The Ottawa Hospital, Ottawa, Ontario, Canada

EVAN SIAU, MD
Hospitalist, Department of Medicine, Mount Sinai Beth Israel, Clinical Instructor, Icahn School of Medicine at Mount Sinai, New York, New York, USA

BRAGHADHEESWAR THYAGARAJAN, MD
Fellow, Department of Anesthesiology, Section on Critical Care Medicine, Wake Forest School of Medicine, Wake Forest Baptist Medical Center, Winston-Salem, North Carolina, USA

LINDA WANG, MD
Assistant Professor, Division of General Internal Medicine, Department of Medicine, Icahn School of Medicine at Mount Sinai, New York, New York, USA

STACEY-ANN WHITTAKER BROWN, MD, MPH
Division of Pulmonary, Critical Care and Sleep Medicine, Icahn School of Medicine at Mount Sinai, New York, New York, USA

JEFF WIESE, MD
Professor of Medicine, Department of Internal Medicine, Tulane University, New Orleans, Louisiana, USA

Contents

Sepsis and Septic Shock – Basics of diagnosis, pathophysiology and clinical decision making   573

Michael D. Font, Braghadheeswar Thyagarajan, and Ashish K. Khanna

> Sepsis and septic shock are major causes of mortality among hospitalized patients. The sepsis state is due to dysregulated host response to infection, leading to inflammatory damage to nearly every organ system. Early recognition of sepsis and appropriate treatment with antibiotics, fluids, and vasopressors is essential to reducing organ system injury and mortality. This review summarizes the current understanding of the epidemiology, pathophysiology, diagnosis, and treatment of sepsis and septic shock.

Management of Pneumonia Syndromes in the Hospital: Make Pneumonia Your Best Friend   587

Abraham Kanal, Bradley A. Sharpe, and Jesse Abelson

> Pneumonia syndromes are defined as acute infections of the pulmonary parenchyma. Pneumonia syndromes continue to cause substantial morbidity and mortality in the hospital. Common syndromes faced by hospital-based providers include: community-acquired pneumonia, hospital-acquired pneumonia, ventilator-associated pneumonia, and aspiration pneumonitis/pneumonia. Substantial evidence and guidelines have provided evidence-based recommendations on the diagnosis and treatment of these syndromes. Future research will provide more insight into the microbiology, optimal diagnostic testing, and best therapeutic options for these syndromes. This article provides a comprehensive review of the common pneumonia syndromes with a particular focus on community-acquired pneumonia.

Advances in the Management of Acute Decompensated Heart Failure   601

Sumeet S. Mitter and Sean P. Pinney

> Patients hospitalized for heart failure pose a considerable clinical and financial burden on the health care system. Early recognition and deep phenotyping of heart failure for reduced and preserved ejection fraction syndromes facilitate the introduction of appropriate guideline-directed therapy and decongestion strategies to help improve heart failure morbidity and mortality. Robust and safe transitions of care programs are needed to deliver adequate care and improve overall survival.

Chronic obstructive pulmonary disease is a chronic, irreversible obstructive lung disease that results from exposure to noxious stimuli. Acute exacerbations of chronic obstructive pulmonary disease (AECOPD) usually result from viral or bacterial respiratory infections, but may also result from exposure to environmental pollution. AECOPD are associated with functional decline, increased risk of subsequent exacerbations, and death. Despite the poor prognosis of AECOPD, patients are empowered through self-management programs in their battle against this lethal disease. Morbidity and mortality can be reduced by implementing standardized treatment modalities outlined in this article throughout the hospitalization and beyond.

Acute venous thromboembolism is a common disease seen by nearly all hospitalists. The advent of low molecular weight heparin (LMWH) several decades ago ushered in the era of early hospital discharge and home treatment. More recently, the direct oral anticoagulants (DOACs) have further simplified outpatient treatment and some offer treatment without parenteral therapy. Use of DOACs for cancer-associated venous thromboembolism is emerging and is a welcome evolution of care to spare oncologic patients the burden of daily LMWH injections.

Hospitalists often care for patients with liver disease, including those with acute liver injury and failure and patients with complications of decompensated cirrhosis. Acute liver failure is a true emergency, requiring intensive care and oftentimes transfer of the patient to a liver transplant center. Patients with decompensated cirrhosis have complications of portal hypertension, including variceal hemorrhage, ascites, spontaneous bacterial peritonitis, and hepatic encephalopathy. These complications increase the risk of mortality among patients with decompensated cirrhosis. Comanagement by the hospitalist with gastroenterology/hepatology can optimize care, especially for patients being considered for liver transplant evaluation.

Hospital-acquired infections increase cost, morbidity, and mortality for patients across the United States and the world. Principal among these infections are central line–associated bloodstream infection, catheter-associated urinary tract infection, Clostridioides difficile, and methicillin-resistant Staphylococcus aureus colonization and infections. This article provides succinct summaries of the background, epidemiology, diagnosis, and treatment of these conditions. In addition, novel prevention strategies, including those related to recent national interventions, are reviewed.

Alcohol use is a common social and recreational activity in our society. Misuse of alcohol can lead to significant medical comorbidities that can affect essentially every organ system and lead to high health care costs and utilization. Heavy alcohol use across the spectrum from binge drinking and intoxication to chronic alcohol use disorder can lead to high morbidity and mortality both in the long and short term. Recognizing and treating common neurologic, gastrointestinal, and hematological manifestations of excess alcohol intake are essential for those who care for hospitalized patients. Withdrawal is among the most common and dangerous sequela associated with alcohol use disorder.

The diagnosis of opioid use disorder (OUD) is often overlooked or inadequately managed during the inpatient admission. When recognized, a common strategy is opioid detoxification, an approach that is often ineffective and can be potentially dangerous because of loss of tolerance and subsequent risk for overdose. Medication for addiction treatment (MAT), including methadone and buprenorphine, is effective and can be dispensed in the hospital for both opioid withdrawal and initiation of maintenance treatment. Hospitalists should be knowledgeable about diagnosing and managing patients with OUD, including how to manage acute pain or MAT during the perioperative setting.

Decisions surrounding periprocedural anticoagulation management must balance thromboembolic and procedural bleed risk. The interruption of both warfarin and DOACs requires consideration of anticoagulant pharmacokinetics, procedural bleed risk and patient characteristics. There is a diminishing role for periprocedural bridging LMWH overall and no role for bridging LMWH for the procedural interruption of DOACs. A clinical approach to perioperative DOAC management based on operative bleeding risk and renal function is safe and effective, and at present, is preferred over preprocedural DOAC levels testing. Clear communication of the anticoagulation interruption plan to both the patient and the patient's care team is essential.

> Teamwork is essential to providing high-quality patient care. Hospital settings pose important challenges to teamwork. Measurement is key to understanding baseline performance and assessing whether teamwork is improving. The authors recommend a multifaceted approach, using a combination of complementary interventions with an ultimate goal that improved teamwork translates into improved patient outcomes.

> Although not suitable for every patient encounter, rounding at the beside provides an opportunity to teach and augment the attitudes essential for optimal medical care. It also provides an opportunity to establish and grow the team's culture as well as the culture for each patient encounter. Finally, it provides the attending physician with an opportunity to assess learners' position on the supervision-to-autonomy spectrum, thereby ensuring appropriate supervision while enabling the autonomy necessary for optimal learner growth.

Foreword
All Medicine Is Local

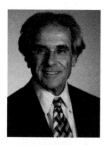

Jack Ende, MD, MACP
Consulting Editor

The famed Boston politician and Speaker of the House of Representatives, Tip O'Neill, is often credited with the admonition, "All politics is local." Tip was right! What works politically in one environment may not necessarily work in another.

But what about medicine? Can rules, lessons, and trusted algorithms developed for one environment, the office, for example, be applied to another, specifically the hospital? Your faithful Consulting Editor, who has always practiced in both environments, primarily the office, but also the hospital, says NO, they cannot, or at least not without modification. And why is that?

First, because the exigencies of hospital medicine have changed and will not change back. Gone are the days when patients with nephrotic syndrome would be admitted to the hospital, started on steroids, and monitored in the hospital for weeks on end, until a significant reduction in proteinuria could be documented. I need not describe how different things are now.

Second, because the demands on the office-based primary care physician (PCP) have also significantly changed. Whether due to changes in reimbursement, patient demand, or simply the understandable desire for a saner schedule, most office-based PCPs no longer can (and many believe no long should) round in the hospital.

And third, in so many ways, hospital care has become much more complex. Ventilator management, discharge planning, antibiotic selection, and attention to patient safety, all call for special expertise. Hospital-based physicians need to be familiar not only with the rudiments but also with the intricacies and nuances of hospital care. Extrapolation from the office no longer will do.

I, for one, take this as a positive step, a step along the same path physicians have always followed. Internists and other providers have always put the needs of patients first. Now, we need to appreciate that our patients in the hospital have special needs. And so it was with great enthusiasm that I recruited Dr Andrew Dunn to take on the role of Guest Editor and provide for the *Medical Clinics of North America* with this volume

Med Clin N Am 104 (2020) xv–xvi
https://doi.org/10.1016/j.mcna.2020.04.002
0025-7125/20/© 2020 Published by Elsevier Inc.

an update on Hospitalist Medicine. The issue he and his authors have produced is outstanding. It covers important topics in acute illness, including septic shock, pneumonia, heart failure, chronic obstructive pulmonary disease, and cirrhosis, and illness related to alcohol and substance abuse. It also covers complications associated with hospitalization perioperative management and, finally, teamwork and teaching. These articles are of great interest to hospitalists, of course, but also to PCPs who need to understand the hospital care their patients receive.

Colleagues, we are past the point of wondering whether hospitalist medicine deserves a place at the table. It does. And we and our patients will benefit as a result. I hope you are able to invest precious study time in this volume of *Medical Clinics of North America*. You will find a trove of medical wisdom assembled by authors who have lent their expertise to bringing us all up-to-date.

Jack Ende, MD, MACP
The Schaeffer Professor of Medicine
Perelman School of Medicine of
the University of Pennsylvania
5033 W. Gates Pavilion
3400 Spruce Street
Philadelphia, PA 19104, USA

E-mail address:
jack.ende@uphs.upenn.edu

Preface

Realizing the Potential of Hospitalist Medicine

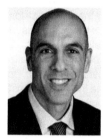

Andrew S. Dunn, MD, MPH, SFHM, MACP
Editor

The bar to break even is high, and the goal is not to break even. Hospital medicine has been the fastest growing field in medicine due to multiple factors; none of which are a proven net benefit over the traditional model when the posthospitalization period is considered. A traditional model, which can also be called "historic" in recognition of its current impracticality and rarity, here refers to a primary care physician (PCP) who sees a patient longitudinally over years, provides care as the attending of record while the patient is hospitalized, and seamlessly resumes outpatient care promptly after discharge. It's hard to argue with the intuitive benefits of the approach.

Kuo and Goodwin[1] provided the initial evidence for the comparison between hospitalists and pcps. They sampled 5% of us medicare patients who were hospitalized and compared outcomes based on the assigned attending. The analysis adjusted for baseline differences between groups through application of a propensity score to a logistic regression model. The study found that patients cared for by hospitalists had shorter length of stay (LOS) and lower hospital charges than patients cared for by their pcp, though patients cared for by their pcp had fewer emergency department visits, fewer readmissions, were more likely to be discharged directly home, and had lower cost in the 30 days after hospitalization than patients cared for by hospitalists.

A larger study by stevens and colleagues[2] shed further light on the different outcomes that may result based on the field of the inpatient physician. These investigators examined over 560,000 medicare admissions and categorized patients as being cared for by their outpatient pcp, a hospitalist, or other generalist (ie, a non-pcp, non–hospitalist physician). The results again demonstrated that PCPs set the standard for outcomes extending beyond the walls of the hospital. Patients cared for by their pcp had higher LOS but were less likely to be discharged to a skilled nursing facility and had lower 30-day mortality than patients cared for by a hospitalist. Notably, only 14% of patients in this national sample were cared for by their pcp during their

Med Clin N Am 104 (2020) xvii–xx
https://doi.org/10.1016/j.mcna.2020.04.001
0025-7125/20/© 2020 Elsevier Inc. All rights reserved.

hospitalization, highlighting the difficulties pcps face in providing care for their patients when hospitalized. The study also helps elucidate the impact on patient care and outcomes had a hospitalist model not evolved. Compared with other generalists, patients cared for by hospitalists had lower los, were more likely to be discharged home, had fewer readmissions, and had decreased mortality. Hospitalists are clearly providing tremendous value to patients and hospitals.

These studies have limitations. Most notably, the nonrandomized designs may have yielded a sicker population in the hospitalist groups that may not have been fully adjusted for by the logistical analyses. However, taken together, these studies provide the best available evidence of the benefits and challenges of the hospitalist model. The experience, expertise, and focus of career-oriented hospitalists provide benefit for patients while hospitalized and improve important outcomes beyond hospitalization relative to non-pcp physicians. A model where the pcp provides care for hospitalized patients provides the best net outcomes when including the immediate post-hospitalization period.

As hospitalists, we need to aspire to match or surpass the outcomes that can be achieved by a pcp-only model. However, more than individual commitment is needed for the promise of the hospitalist model to be achieved; hospitals and hospital medicine practices need to provide the support and structure for optimal outcomes to be realized. Important components of any group's plan to improve performance will be retention, development, and a commitment to communication.

Retention is essential for the success of any hospitalist practice. A hospitalist model where physicians cycle through positions does not allow development of the intrahospital relationships, teamwork skills, and expertise required to deliver optimal performance. In his book, "Outliers," Malcolm Gladwell made popular the notion that 10,000 hours of practice are required for expertise in a field or craft to develop.[3] The theory originated in a 1993 paper by psychologist anders ericcson that suggested that 10 years are required for expert performance.[4] The "10,000-hour rule" has since generated substantial discussion and debate, including over the contribution of innate talent. In addition, it is important to recognize that 10,000 is an average rather than a fixed value. Most relevantly, time needs to be spent in "deliberate practice" rather than simply marking the passing of time. The concept suggests that patients and hospitals greatly benefit by having hospitalists dedicated to lifelong learning working in an environment that promotes development, and that these efforts do not reach fruition for several years. As retention is essential for group success, attention and resources need to focus on areas that will provide a sustainable and nourishing work environment. These efforts should address adequate schedule flexibility, attention to work-life balance, providing meaning in work, opportunities for development and advancement, and fostering community among team members.

Retaining physicians will be a hollow accomplishment without attention to development. The "deliberate practice" framework has direct relevance to hospitalists. A deliberate process that includes an active learning environment will greatly increase the yield in knowledge and skills relative to purely passive processes. As an example, regularly reflecting on clinical decisions, the decision-making process, and outcomes provides tremendous opportunity to expand the knowledge base and illness scripts. Such moments can be great sources of growth, whether considering a diagnosis that was missed or an uncommon diagnosis made promptly.

Explicit efforts in lifelong learning are challenging given the extraordinary workload faced by physicians, though well worth the effort when the right sources are chosen. Reading this issue of the *Medical Clinics of North America* is a great start. The authors are nationally renowned experts who have provided highly valuable content on core topics, including congestive heart failure, venous thromboembolism, and teamwork. Busy physicians should also avail themselves of other formats and modalities that best suit their time available and learning needs. Many are fun and invigorating. Some suggestions and examples include the following:

- Podcasts: several podcasts focus on clinical decision making through case discussion as small aliquots of information are revealed.
- Apps: the human diagnosis app provides brief, challenging case presentations with an opportunity to provide a differential diagnosis, and a set of teaching pearls after the diagnosis is revealed.
- Clinical case presentations: read along with the case presentations in major medical journals. A key to increase your yield is to generate your own clinical thinking before you read each set of expert discussant comments.
- Interactive web-based educational modules: many specialty societies offer valuable web-based content. The american college of physicians web site's online learning center has interactive cases, modules on management of opioid use disorder, point-of-care ultrasound, and numerous other topics.
- Tweetorials:these are sequences of twitter posts from expert clinicians that provide concise pearls that progress over a series. Physicians who seek content in a fast-paced and potentially interactive format may find tweetorials valuable.

These are just a few examples of the increasingly innovative and varied content that are available to physicians motivated to develop their expertise. Readers are encouraged to find the formats and venues that they find the most fun and feasible and make these educational activities a routine part of their schedule.

Retaining and developing hospitalists are essential strategies to achieving outstanding outcomes. However, regardless of the expertise, there remains an inevitable loss of information from having greater than 1 physician involved in care.[5] The clear gains from a hospitalist model that occur during hospitalization can be negated by a suboptimal transition of care.[6] One potential solution is to ask hospitalists to commit to routine communication with the outpatient physician. This approach is likely to fail. Most hospitalists are already striving to communicate and provide excellent care. Asking physicians to "work harder" produces little long-term improvement. Rather, systems need to be developed to help remove barriers and promote a culture of communication. Ideally, this includes a shared electronic medical record (EMR). A shared emr can provide the pcp with automated notification of admissions and discharges; can provide access to notes, including the discharge summary; and can facilitate interprofessional communication, such as through emr-based secure text messages.

Communication between inpatient and outpatient physicians who are not using a shared emr is more challenging.[7,8] processes that may facilitate communication can include structured admission templates or orders that include the name and contact information of the pcp, and having this information prominently displayed on all emr patient lists. Structured processes that send discharge summaries to outpatient physicians will enhance communication without imposing a clerical task on the hospitalists. A more burdensome system requires documentation of communication, or the attempt at communication, by the inpatient physician in an auditable field. However, it is far from assured that such a system will improve patient care. Whether the yield is worth the burden needs to be determined locally; adding tasks with little or no proven benefit impedes patient care.

The journey to deliver on the promise of hospital medicine is challenging yet inspiring. I am glad to be able to share the road with so many colleagues with similar interests and aspirations. The authors and i hope you will find this issue valuable on your path.

Andrew S. Dunn, MD, MPH, SFHM, MACP
Division of Hospital Medicine
Mount Sinai Health System
1468 Madison Avenue, Box 1086
New York, NY 10029, USA

E-mail address:
andrew.dunn@mountsinai.org

REFERENCES

1. Kuo YF, Goodwin JS. Association of hospitalist care with medical utilization after discharge: evidence of cost shift from a cohort study. Ann Int Med 2011;155: 152–9.
2. Stevens JP, Nyweide DJ, Maresh S, et al. Comparison of hospital resource use and outcomes among hospitalists, primary care physicians, and other generalists. JAMA Int Med 2017;177:1781–7.
3. Gladwell M. Outliers: the story of success. New York: Back Bay Books; 2011.
4. Ericsson A. The role of deliberate practice in the acquisition of expert performance. Psychol Rev 1993;100:363–406.
5. Jones CD, Vu MB, O'Donnell CM, et al. A failure to communicate: a qualitative exploration of care coordination between hospitalists and primary care providers around patient hospitalizations. J Gen Int Med 2015;30:417–24.
6. Moore CM, Wisnivesky J, Williams S, et al. Medical errors related to discontinuity of care from an inpatient to an outpatient setting. J Gen Int Med 2003;18:646–51.
7. Hesselink P, Schoohoven L, Barach P, et al. Improving patient handovers from hospital to primary care: a systematic review. Ann Intern Med 2012;157:417–28.
8. Kripalani S, Jackson AT, Schnipper JL, et al. Promoting effective transitions of care at hospital discharge: a review of key issues for hospitalists. J Hosp Med 2007;2: 314–23.

Sepsis and Septic Shock – Basics of diagnosis, pathophysiology and clinical decision making

Michael D. Font, MD[a], Braghadheeswar Thyagarajan, MD[b],
Ashish K. Khanna, MD, FCCP, FCCM[b,c],*

KEYWORDS

- Critical care • Sepsis • Septic shock • SIRS • qSOFA • Vasopressors

KEY POINTS

- The definition of sepsis has evolved over time. Most recently, the term "sepsis" has been defined as life-threatening organ dysfunction caused by a dysregulated host response to infection.
- There are several screening tools available to identify sepsis, including the SIRS (Systemic Inflammatory Response Syndrome) criteria and the qSOFA (quick Sequential Organ Failure Assessment) score. These tools have imperfect sensitivity and specificity and should be used carefully.
- The septic state affects nearly every organ system and can lead to profound derangements in physiology and laboratory findings.
- Management of sepsis relies on early identification and empiric antimicrobial therapy, adequate but not excessive fluid resuscitation, and support of hemodynamic goals with vasopressors.
- Several classes of vasopressors are available, including catecholamines, vasopressin, and renin-angiotensin-aldosterone agonists. Norepinephrine has been suggested as the initial vasopressor of choice; however, multimodal vasopressor therapy may be useful to avoid deleterious effects of high-dose monotherapy.

INTRODUCTION

As of 2017, the World Health Organization has made the recognition, prevention, and management of sepsis a global health priority.[1] Hippocrates considered the term

[a] Department of Anesthesiology, Wake Forest School of Medicine, Wake Forest Baptist Medical Center, 1, Medical Center Boulevard, Winston-Salem, NC 27157, USA; [b] Department of Anesthesiology, Section on Critical Care Medicine, Wake Forest School of Medicine, Wake Forest Baptist Medical Center, 1, Medical Center Boulevard, Winston-Salem, NC 27157, USA; [c] Outcomes Research Consortium, Cleveland, OH 44195, USA
* Corresponding author. Outcomes Research Consortium, Cleveland, OH 44195.
E-mail address: akhanna@wakehealth.edu

Med Clin N Am 104 (2020) 573–585
https://doi.org/10.1016/j.mcna.2020.02.011
0025-7125/20/© 2020 Elsevier Inc. All rights reserved.

"sepsis" as a process of rotting flesh, and recently, it has been defined as life-threatening organ dysfunction resulting from infection.[1] Despite best efforts at protocol-based care pathways, mortality from septic shock remains high at nearly 35% to 40%.[2]

Sepsis-1: Systemic Inflammatory Response Syndrome Criteria

The term "sepsis" had been used broadly for decades; however, it had been associated with multiple definitions, and the term had been loosely applied to many syndromes. In an effort to improve the ability to study sepsis, a convention of experts met in 1992 and formalized the definition of the term.[3] At that time, the term "sepsis" was defined as an inflammatory response to infection. The clinical diagnosis was defined by 2 or more Systemic Inflammatory Response Syndrome (SIRS) criteria paired with a suspected or confirmed source of infection.[4] Septic shock was defined at this time as persistent hypotension or hyperlactatemia despite fluid resuscitation.

Sepsis 2.0 and "Severe Sepsis"

Many criticisms arose regarding the Sepsis-1 definitions, most notably that the SIRS criteria merely reflected an appropriate response to infection. A new term had emerged, "severe sepsis," which implied organ dysfunction as a result of the sepsis state. In 2001, a second expert group convened to update the Sepsis-1 definitions.[5] The definitions were left largely unchanged, with the exception of the introduction of the Sequential Organ Failure Assessment (SOFA) criteria to identify organ dysfunction, which was indicative of severe sepsis (**Table 1**).

2016 Update: Sepsis 3.0

The initial definition specified in the Sepsis-1 criteria was widely used for almost 2 - decades; however, it was hindered by poor sensitivity and specificity. A main criticism is that the physiology implied by the SIRS criteria (tachycardia, fever, leukocytosis, and hypotension) are focused on the inflammatory response, which is common to many critical illnesses (trauma, pancreatitis, postsurgical inflammation).[6] To illustrate, more than 90% of patients admitted to an intensive care unit (ICU) met the criteria for sepsis.[7] Another criticism is that the SIRS criteria failed to identify 13% of patients with similar profiles of infection, organ failure, and substantially increased mortality.[8]

Table 1
Comparison of older and new definitions for the spectrum of sepsis and septic shock

	Sepsis-2 Definitions	Sepsis 3.0 Definitions
Sepsis	≥2 SIRS criteria AND Suspected infection	Increase in SOFA score ≥2 from baseline OR qSOFA ≥2 AND Suspected infection
Severe sepsis	Sepsis AND Organ dysfunction (change in SOFA ≥2 points)	(Not applicable)
Septic shock	Sepsis AND Hypotension despite fluid resuscitation OR Lactatemia despite fluid resuscitation	Sepsis AND Vasopressor requirement despite fluid resuscitation OR Lactate >2 mmol/L after resuscitation

Because the inflammatory response is an expected and useful response in many cases of infection, a challenge for a new definition of sepsis was to differentiate the life-threatening, dysregulated response present with sepsis from the normal inflammatory response of uncomplicated infection. In 2016, the Sepsis Task Force again updated the definition to be the pattern of life-threatening organ dysfunction caused by a dysregulated host response to infection.[9]

Clinically, this was characterized by an acute change of 2 or more points in the SOFA score in the setting of suspicion for infection.[9,10] The baseline score is assumed to be 0 in patients not known to have preexisting organ dysfunction. The SOFA score had a good predictive validity for mortality of patients in the ICU. For patients with suspected infection, the area under the receiver operating characteristic (AUROC) is 0.74. This number is superior to the SIRS criteria, which has an AUROC of 0.66.[9]

Under this new definition, the term "severe sepsis" is redundant. Accordingly, this term was dropped from the updated definition. Septic shock was defined as the subset of sepsis with profound circulatory, cellular, and metabolic dysregulation, and associated with a much higher mortality of ~40%, compared with the 10% mortality observed with sepsis.[9,11] Septic shock is clinically identified as a persistent hypotension requiring vasopressors to keep mean arterial pressure (MAP) greater than 65 mm Hg and elevated serum lactate greater than 2 mmol/L, *despite* adequate fluid resuscitation.

Quick Sequential Organ Failure Assessment Screening Tool

Although the change in SOFA score is a robust mortality stratification tool, it is cumbersome to calculate and requires laboratory values that are not readily available for quick screening of patients outside of the ICU. For example, a serum lactate level that is routinely analyzed from a blood gas sample in the ICU may be difficult to do on a ward patient and on a serial basis. The task force set out to identify readily accessible screening measures and arrived at 3 criteria, termed the qSOFA (quick Sequential Organ Failure Assessment). For patients outside of the ICU who had 2 or more of the following criteria: Glasgow score less than 13, systolic blood pressure less than 100 or respiratory rate (RR) $\geq$22, mortality was similar to those patients identified using the full SOFA score.[9]

Performance of Quick Sequential Organ Failure Assessment Versus Sequential Organ Failure Assessment Versus Systemic Inflammatory Response Syndrome for Screening

Subsequent studies have highlighted the need for careful use of the tools for different patient populations. As a screening tool for emergency department (ED) patients, multiple studies have shown worse performance of qSOFA compared with SIRS for early identification of sepsis.[12–14] As a prognostic risk stratification tool of ICU patients, the SOFA score better predicted mortality.[14] A systematic review found similar results; the SIRS criteria had better sensitivity but worsened specificity for the detection of sepsis among ED, ICU, and hospital wards patients.[15]

EPIDEMIOLOGY

In the United States, there are currently ~1.7 million cases of sepsis per year, a trend that has been increasing annually. There are almost 250,000 deaths per year owing to sepsis, and it is the leading cause of death in noncardiac ICUs.[16,17]

Of septic patients admitted to ICUs worldwide, the most common source of infection is the lungs (64%), abdomen (20%), bloodstream (15%), and urinary tract (14%).

Of isolated organisms, 62% were gram-negative bacteria; 47% were gram-positive bacteria, and 19% were fungi.[17]

The most common gram-positive organism is *Staphylococcus aureus* (20%), and the most common gram-negative isolates are *Pseudomonas* (20%) and *Escherichia coli* (16%).[17]

Many factors are associated with increased risk of mortality in patients with sepsis and septic shock: emergency surgery (odds ratio [OR] 1.56), trauma (OR 1.01), transfer from hospital floor (OR 1.37), presence of chronic obstructive pulmonary disease (OR 1.21), cancer (OR 1.33), heart failure (OR 1.45), immunosuppression (OR 1.81), cirrhosis (OR 2.14), previous mechanical ventilation (OR 1.90), or hemodialysis (OR 1.58).[17]

PATHOPHYSIOLOGY

The pathophysiology underlying the septic state is complex. It is unclear why some patients mount a productive immune response to fight infection, whereas others deteriorate into a dysregulated state. The role of several cellular mediators has been investigated, especially tumor necrosis factor-α and interleukin-1, which can reproduce the sepsis symptoms when administered exogenously.[18,19] It was previously thought that sepsis was the result of a "cytokine storm" of these mediators; however, it has since been shown that release of proinflammatory mediators is also accompanied by anti-inflammatory mediators.[20,21]

It is also known that exogenous administration of lipopolysaccharide (LPS) leads to endothelial damage and shedding of the endothelial glycocalyx. This mechanism leads to the hyperpermeability and edema formation that are seen with sepsis.[22] LPS also causes the release of nitric oxide (NO) from damaged endothelial cells, which leads to pathologic arteriodilation and hypoperfusion. Conversely, exogenous inducible nitric oxide synthase inhibitors appear to reverse the pathologic vasodilation in animal models.[23]

CLINICAL MANIFESTATIONS BY ORGAN SYSTEM

The presenting signs and symptoms of sepsis often involve multiple organ systems. Profound release of various inflammatory mediators during sepsis leads to multiorgan system failure (**Fig. 1**). Hence, sepsis needs to be managed as a systemic disorder.

Cardiovascular

Pathologic arterial and venodilation leads to hypotension, which can be profound. In addition, myocardial depression is observed in up to 60% of septic patients.[24] The exact mechanism of this septic cardiomyopathy is unclear. Mildly elevated troponin levels are commonly observed and can be linked to severity of sepsis.[25]

Pulmonary

Cytokine-mediated lung injury results in increased permeability of alveolar and capillary endothelium, causing noncardiogenic pulmonary edema, which impairs oxygenation and ventilation.[26] Development of hypoxia and metabolic acidosis results in significant tachypnea. The incidence of acute respiratory distress syndrome (ARDS) in patients with sepsis is 7%.[27] Careful monitoring of respiratory parameters is key in identifying patients who will require intubation and mechanical ventilation because of respiratory muscle fatigue.[25]

Renal

Sepsis-related acute kidney injury (AKI) contributes significantly to morbidity and mortality of sepsis.[28] Risk factors for the development of AKI are advanced age,

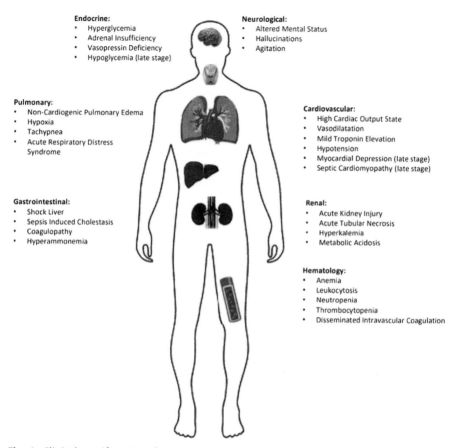

Endocrine:
- Hyperglycemia
- Adrenal Insufficiency
- Vasopressin Deficiency
- Hypoglycemia (late stage)

Neurological:
- Altered Mental Status
- Hallucinations
- Agitation

Pulmonary:
- Non-Cardiogenic Pulmonary Edema
- Hypoxia
- Tachypnea
- Acute Respiratory Distress Syndrome

Cardiovascular:
- High Cardiac Output State
- Vasodilatation
- Mild Troponin Elevation
- Hypotension
- Myocardial Depression (late stage)
- Septic Cardiomyopathy (late stage)

Gastrointestinal:
- Shock Liver
- Sepsis Induced Cholestasis
- Coagulopathy
- Hyperammonemia

Renal:
- Acute Kidney Injury
- Acute Tubular Necrosis
- Hyperkalemia
- Metabolic Acidosis

Hematology:
- Anemia
- Leukocytosis
- Neutropenia
- Thrombocytopenia
- Disseminated Intravascular Coagulation

Fig. 1. Clinical manifestations by organ system.

chronic kidney disease, and cardiovascular disease.[29] The pathophysiology is multifactorial, including hemodynamic changes, endothelial dysfunction, inflammation of the renal parenchyma, and obstruction of tubules with necrotic cells and debris.[30] Prompt volume resuscitation, preventing hypotension and avoiding the use of nephrotoxic agents, such as intravenous contrast, can help mitigate the risks of developing AKI. Once AKI has developed, appropriate dosing of medications, avoiding volume overload by the use of diuretics, and careful management of electrolytes are required.[31] In patients requiring renal replacement therapy, there appears to be benefit to early initiation over delayed initiation.[32]

Hematological

The primary hematological manifestations are anemia, leukocytosis, neutropenia, thrombocytopenia, and disseminated intravascular coagulation (DIC).[33] Inhibition of thrombopoiesis and immunologic platelet damage are responsible for the thrombocytopenia observed without DIC.[34] Anemia is secondary to inflammation, shortened red blood cell survival, and hemolysis in the setting of DIC. DIC is diagnosed by thrombocytopenia, and prolongation of prothrombin time or activated partial thromboplastin time. DIC in sepsis can present as bleeding from multiple sites or thrombosis of small and medium blood vessels. In the absence of bleeding, coagulopathy can be monitored along with treatment of underlying disorder. In patients with bleeding from multiple sites, platelet and coagulation factor replacement should be considered.[33]

Gastrointestinal

Liver failure is an uncommon but significant complication of septic shock, occurring in less than 2% of septic patients, with a marked impact on morbidity and mortality.[35] Septic hepatic dysfunction is diagnosed by an increase in bilirubin concentration greater than 2 mg/dL and coagulopathy with international normalized ratio greater than 1.5.[36] The pathophysiology is attributed to hemodynamic, cellular, molecular, and immunologic changes leading to parenchymal hypoxia. Clinical manifestations include hypoxic hepatitis, sepsis-induced cholestasis, coagulopathies, and hyperammonemia, causing hepatic encephalopathy.[37]

Endocrine

Hyperglycemia is common in septic patients and is attributed to stress-induced elevation of glucagon, catecholamines, cortisol, and growth hormone–combined insulin resistance induced by the release of cytokines.[38] Glucose should be frequently monitored in septic shock, with the goal of keeping blood glucose less than 180 mg/dL, while avoiding overaggressive control and associated hypoglycemic episodes.[36] In addition to metabolic dysregulation, 8% to 9% of patients with severe sepsis have evidence of adrenal insufficiency, which can further contribute to catecholamine insensitivity.[39] Management with exogenous steroids is discussed separately. Septic patients also have vasopressin deficiency due to depletion of stores, increased vasopressinase activity, and nitric oxide–mediated inhibition of vasopressin production.[40] The hypothalamic-pituitary-thyroid axis can also be affected during sepsis, leading to apparent clinical hypothyroidism; however, there is no evidence favoring the treatment of septic hypothyroidism.[38,41]

Neurologic

Septic encephalopathy is a common manifestation of severe sepsis and septic shock. Symptoms can include changes in mental status, alteration in sleep/wake cycle, disorientation, agitation, and hallucinations. Altered mental status may be the only presenting sign in geriatric patients. Focal deficits are not typical of septic encephalopathy and should be evaluated with neuroimaging and stroke workup. Seizure is a rare complication of septic encephalopathy and may be diagnosed with electroencephalographic monitoring.[42] In the event of significant alterations in mental status, some patients may require endotracheal intubation for airway protection. Other reversible causes of encephalopathy, such as hypoxemia, hypercapnia, hypoglycemia, hyponatremia or hypernatremia, drug toxicity, hyperammonemia, and thyroid insufficiency, should to be rapidly assessed and ruled out.[25]

MANAGEMENT OF SEPSIS AND SEPTIC SHOCK
Era of Early Goal-Directed Therapy

In 2001, a landmark trial was published that demonstrated mortality benefit to "early goal-directed therapy" (EGDT), which used an algorithm of fluid resuscitation, blood transfusion, vasopressors, and inotropes to targeted specific hemodynamic goals of MAP, central venous pressure, and mixed venous oxygen saturation.[43] This trial ushered in an era of sepsis care in which pulmonary artery catheters were routinely placed in most septic patients to monitor these parameters.

More recent trials have failed to replicate the results of EGDT, and the practice of algorithmic resuscitation has mostly fallen out of favor.[44–46] However, many of the principles of fluid resuscitation and hemodynamic goals still remain in place and are reflected in the Surviving Sepsis Campaign guidelines.[36]

Screening and Diagnosis

If concern for sepsis is elevated based on screening criteria (qSOFA or SIRS) and clinical picture, initial management should not be delayed while awaiting further diagnostic studies. Blood cultures should be drawn promptly, and urine cultures should be collected if there is suspicion for urinary tract infection. Imaging should usually include a chest X ray to rule out developing pneumonia, and further imaging, such as abdominal computed tomographic scan if there is suspicion for intraabdominal process (eg, diverticulitis, abscess). Procalcitonin levels may be drawn early in the process, not to act as a diagnostic criterion, but to later guide antibiotic cessation for certain infections.[47]

Antibiotics and Source Control

Observational studies have suggested that early initiation of antibiotic therapy may be associated with better outcomes, and this idea has been incorporated into the Surviving Sepsis Guidelines as a goal of initiation of antibiotics within 1 hour of presentation.[48] There is concern that these data are not robust, and that this guideline will lead to widespread inappropriate utilization of antibiotics.[49]

When there is adequate suspicion for sepsis, cultures should be obtained and broad-spectrum antibiotic therapy should be initiated to empirically cover a range of likely pathogens, dependent on the patient's comorbidities and presentation. In most patients, antibiotics should be directed toward gram-positive and gram-negative bacteria. In patients with an intraabdominal process, anaerobic coverage is indicated. In patients with immunodeficiencies or immunosuppression, antifungal and/or antiviral therapies may be indicated.

The antimicrobial therapy should be narrowed based on the results of cultures, as able. Serial procalcitonin measurements have been shown to successfully guide cessation of antibiotic therapy to reduce cumulative exposure.[47]

The source of the infection should be addressed if possible. The patient should be closely examined for a localized source, such as infected pressure ulcer or erythematous vascular catheter site. Management may include removal of invasive devices (eg, dialysis catheters, infected orthopedic hardware, or pacemakers) or surgical evacuation of intraabdominal abscess.

Fluid Resuscitation

Observational studies have demonstrated that reducing the duration of hypotension in sepsis is associated with decreased mortality in septic shock.[50] The premise of fluid resuscitation is to increase cardiac output and MAP to combat pathologic vasodilation. The Surviving Sepsis Campaign recommends an initial fluid bolus of 30 mL/kg. For most patients, this amount is probably adequate. However, concern has been raised that this volume is probably excessive for many patients. Observational studies have shown that excess volume administration is associated with worsened mortality, which may be due to associated pulmonary edema requiring prolonged mechanical ventilation and worsened kidney injury.[51]

In an effort to avoid overresuscitation, several measures have been used to predict volume-responsiveness, defined as the augmentation of a patient's cardiac output with additional fluid. Bedside echocardiography and ultrasonography have emerged as the most reliable tools, with an increase in the carbon monoxide before and after a "minibolus" of 100 to 250 mL functioning as a reliable indicator.[52,53] The variation of inferior vena cava diameter with inspiration is an accurate predictor of volume responsiveness in mechanically ventilated patients, although there is conflicting evidence in spontaneously breathing patients.[54] Likewise, pulse-pressure variation (PPV) on arterial line tracing can be used under specific conditions with mechanically ventilated patients. For patients who are in sinus rhythm and mechanically ventilated with tidal volumes of greater than 8 mL/kg (ideal body weight), PPV of $\geq$12% is predictive of fluid responsiveness.[55]

Target Blood Pressure

Retrospective data have suggested an association of MAPs less than 85 with progressively increasing risk for mortality and kidney injury.[56,57] The only large randomized trial of 2 blood pressure targets in patients with septic shock attempted to compare the effect of lower MAP target (65–70) compared with higher target (80–85) and did not demonstrate a mortality benefit of one versus the other.[58] However, a prespecified post hoc analysis of the same trial demonstrated significantly increased renal injury in those with preexisting chronic hypertension and maintained at the lower MAP target. On the other hand, there were more cardiac arrhythmias in the higher MAP group, largely because of the likely use of high-dose catecholamines in that arm.[58] Therefore, it may be prudent to maintain relatively higher MAP targets in patients with septic shock, although we are limited by retrospective observational data and cannot recommend a specific threshold that fits all patients.[59,60] Further randomized trials addressing this topic are urgently needed. Of note, the surviving sepsis guidelines recommend a target MAP of at least 65 mm Hg for titrating vasopressor support.[36]

Vasopressor Choice

Vasopressors should be used in septic shock to support the patient's blood pressure during and after fluid resuscitation. Historically, dopamine was recommended as the initial blood pressure agent of choice in septic shock. However, randomized trials comparing the use of dopamine versus norepinephrine as an initial agent showed higher incidences of tachyarrhythmia and worsened mortality with dopamine compared with norepinephrine.[61] Hence, the recommendation from the Surviving Sepsis Campaign that norepinephrine be used as a first-line agent.[62] Epinephrine has been compared with norepinephrine as an initial agent and did not reveal a mortality difference; however, epinephrine was associated with greater tachycardia and lactic acidosis.[63] Specifically, in a septic patient with hypotension and with evidence of cardiomyopathy and associated right heart dysfunction, epinephrine may be added for inotropic benefit and if cardiac output is insufficient to maintain perfusion.[64] Vasopressin is a non–catecholamine molecule that directly acts on V1 and V2 receptors. Vasopressin has also been compared with norepinephrine and showed no mortality benefit overall; however, the subgroup patients with "less severe" septic shock appeared to have slightly lower mortality.[65] In addition to the catecholamine and vasopressin pathways, modulation of the renin-angiotensin-aldosterone pathway has been studied as a means to synergistically augment blood pressure and reduce catecholamine requirements. Exogenous angiotensin II has been shown to increase MAPs and decrease catecholamine requirements in patients with septic shock on high-dose vasopressors and demonstrated a good safety profile.[66] Considering all available current data, norepinephrine remains the first-line agent for initial blood pressure management in septic shock. However, high-dose vasopressors, especially catecholamines at norepinephrine equivalents of 0.8 μg/kg/min or higher, have been associated with a 50% 30-day and almost 80% 90-day mortality.[67] Hence, there is a much-needed push to the early use of multimodal catecholamine-sparing adjunct vasopressors (both vasopressin and angiotensin II) in this regard.[68]

Adjunct Therapies: Steroids, Vitamin C, and Thiamine

Several adjunct therapies have been investigated as mechanisms to combat the body's dysregulated response to sepsis. Systemic steroids have been evaluated in several randomized trials; however, the results of these trials have not consistently demonstrated mortality benefit. Most recently, the ADRENAL trial evaluated the effect of continuous infusion of hydrocortisone on patients with septic shock and did not demonstrate a benefit compared with placebo.[69] The APROCCHSS trial showed modest mortality benefit with the administration of bolus-dose hydrocortisone every 6 hours along with a daily administration of oral fludrocortisone.[70]

Ascorbic acid (vitamin C) has gained attention as an antioxidant that may ameliorate the dysregulated response to sepsis. A small retrospective before-and-after study evaluated the effect of a cocktail of ascorbic acid along with thiamine and hydrocortisone and found promising results.[71] A prospective randomized trial demonstrated decreased vasopressor requirements and decreased mortality in patients receiving bolus-dose ascorbic acid.[72] The CITRIS-ALI trial investigated the role of ascorbic acid on organ dysfunction scores in patients with sepsis and ARDS and showed no significant difference.[73]

SUMMARY

Sepsis and septic shock are leading causes of in-hospital mortality. Sepsis is currently understood as the pattern of life-threatening organ dysfunction caused by a dysregulated host response to infection. Septic shock is the subset of these patients with persistent hypotension and persistently elevated lactate, which is associated with much higher mortality. The SIRS and qSOFA scores can be used to screen patients for sepsis; however, the SIRS tool is associated with poor specificity and the qSOFA score is associated with decreased sensitivity. Initial management of sepsis includes broad-spectrum antimicrobial therapy directed toward likely pathogens, fluid resuscitation guided by measurements of fluid responsiveness, and support of MAP with vasopressors. The initial vasopressor of choice in septic patients is often norepinephrine; however, a multimodal vasopressor regimen using different classes of vasopressors may be required in cases of severe hypotension to avoid the deleterious side effects of escalating 1 vasopressor alone. Adjunct therapies continue to be evaluated for their role in sepsis therapy, including corticosteroids and vitamin supplementation.

DISCLOSURE

Departmental resources supported this work. The authors have nothing to disclose.

REFERENCES

1. Reinhart K, Daniels R, Kissoon N, et al. Recognizing sepsis as a global health priority—a WHO resolution. N Engl J Med 2017;377(5):414–7.

2. Vincent JL, Jones G, David S, et al. Frequency and mortality of septic shock in Europe and North America: a systematic review and meta-analysis. Crit Care 2019. https://doi.org/10.1186/s13054-019-2478-6.

3. American College of Chest Physicians/Society of Critical Care Medicine Consensus Conference: definitions for sepsis and organ failure and guidelines for the use of innovative therapies in sepsis. Crit Care Med 1992. https://doi.org/10.1097/00003246-199206000-00025.

4. Bone RC, Balk RA, Cerra FB, et al. Definitions for sepsis and organ failure and guidelines for the use of innovative therapies in sepsis. Chest 1992;101(6):1644–55.

5. Levy MM, Fink MP, Marshall JC, et al. 2001 SCCM/ESICM/ACCP/ATS/SIS International Sepsis Definitions Conference. Crit Care Med 2003. https://doi.org/10.1097/01.CCM.0000050454.01978.3B.

6. Vincent JL, Opal SM, Marshall JC, et al. Sepsis definitions: time for change. Lancet 2013;381(9868):774–5.

7. Sprung CL, Sakr Y, Vincent JL, et al. An evaluation of systemic inflammatory response syndrome signs in the Sepsis Occurrence in Acutely ill Patients (SOAP) study. Intensive Care Med 2006;32(3):421–7.

8. Kaukonen KM, Bailey M, Pilcher D, et al. Systemic inflammatory response syndrome criteria in defining severe sepsis. N Engl J Med 2015;372(17):1629–38.

9. Singer M, Deutschman CS, Seymour CW, et al. The Third International Consensus definitions for sepsis and septic shock (sepsis-3). JAMA 2016;315(8):801–10.

10. Abraham E. New definitions for sepsis and septic shock. JAMA 2017;114(29–30):801–10.

11. Cecconi M, Evans L, Levy M, et al. Sepsis and septic shock. Lancet 2018;392(10141):75–87.

12. Haydar S, Spanier M, Weems P, et al. Comparison of qSOFA score and SIRS criteria as screening mechanisms for emergency department sepsis. Am J Emerg Med 2017;35(11):1730–3.

13. Usman OA, Usman AA, Ward MA. Comparison of SIRS, qSOFA, and NEWS for the early identification of sepsis in the emergency department. Am J Emerg Med 2018;37(8):1490–7.

14. Raith EP, Udy AA, Bailey M, et al. Prognostic accuracy of the SOFA score, SIRS criteria, and qSOFA score for in-hospital mortality among adults with suspected infection admitted to the intensive care unit. JAMA 2017;317(3):290–300.

15. Fernando SM, Tran A, Taljaard M, et al. Prognostic accuracy of the quick sequential organ failure assessment for mortality in patients with suspected infection: a systematic review and meta-analysis. Ann Intern Med 2018;168(4):266–75.

16. Rhee C, Dantes R, Epstein L, et al. Incidence and trends of sepsis in US hospitals using clinical vs claims data, 2009-2014. JAMA 2017;318(13):1241–9.

17. Vincent JL, Rello J, Marshall J, et al. International study of the prevalence and outcomes of infection in intensive care units. JAMA 2009;302(21):2323–9.

18. Movat HZ, Burrowes CE, Cybulsky MI, et al. Acute inflammation and a Shwartzman-like reaction induced by interleukin-1 and tumor necrosis factor. Synergistic action of the cytokines in the induction of inflammation and microvascular injury. Am J Pathol 1987;129(3):463–76.

19. Dinarello CA, Okusawa S, Gelfand JA. Interleukin-1 induces a shock-like state in rabbits: synergism with tumor necrosis factor and the effect of cyclooxygenase inhibition. Prog Clin Biol Res 1989;286:243–63.

20. Blackwell TS, Christman JW. Sepsis and cytokines: current status. Br J Anaesth 1996;77(1):110–7.

21. Piechota M, Banach M, Irzmanski R, et al. Plasma endothelin-1 levels in septic patients. J Intensive Care Med 2007;22(4):232–9.

22. Ince C, Mayeux PR, Nguyen T, et al. The endothelium in sepsis. Shock 2016; 45(3):259–70.

23. Zhang ZS, Chen W, Li T, et al. Organ-specific changes in vascular reactivity and roles of inducible nitric oxide synthase and endothelin-1 in a rabbit endotoxic shock model. J Trauma Acute Care Surg 2018;85(4):725–33.

24. Vieillard-Baron A, Caille V, Charron C, et al. Actual incidence of global left ventricular hypokinesia in adult septic shock. Crit Care Med 2008;36(6):1701–6.

25. Hotchkiss RS, Moldawer LL, Opal SM, et al. Sepsis and septic shock HHS public access. Nat Rev Dis Primers 2017. https://doi.org/10.1038/nrdp.2016.45.

26. Kim WY, Hong SB. Sepsis and acute respiratory distress syndrome: recent update. Tuberc Respir Dis (Seoul) 2016. https://doi.org/10.4046/trd.2016.79.2.53.

27. Mikkelsen ME, Shah CV, Meyer NJ, et al. The epidemiology of acute respiratory distress syndrome in patients presenting to the emergency department with severe sepsis. Shock 2013. https://doi.org/10.1097/SHK.0b013e3182a64682.

28. Bagshaw SM, Uchino S, Bellomo R, et al. Septic acute kidney injury in critically ill patients: clinical characteristics and outcomes. Clin J Am Soc Nephrol 2007. https://doi.org/10.2215/CJN.03681106.

29. De Mendonça A, Vincent JL, Suter PM, et al. Acute renal failure in the ICU: risk factors and outcome evaluated by the SOFA score. Intensive Care Med 2000. https://doi.org/10.1007/s001340051281.

30. Zarjou A, Agarwal A. Sepsis and acute kidney injury. J Am Soc Nephrol 2011. https://doi.org/10.1681/ASN.2010050484.

31. Godin M, Murray P, Mehta RL. Clinical approach to the patient with AKI and sepsis. Semin Nephrol 2015. https://doi.org/10.1016/j.semnephrol.2015.01.003.

32. Barbar SD, Clere-Jehl R, Bourredjem A, et al. Timing of renal-replacement therapy in patients with acute kidney injury and sepsis. N Engl J Med 2018. https://doi.org/10.1056/NEJMoa1803213.

33. Goyette RE, Key NS, Ely EW. Hematologic changes in sepsis and their therapeutic implications. Semin Respir Crit Care Med 2004. https://doi.org/10.1055/s-2004-860979.

34. Mammen EF. The haematological manifestations of sepsis. J Antimicrob Chemother 1998. https://doi.org/10.1093/jac/41.suppl_1.17.

35. Angus DC, Linde-Zwirble WT, Lidicker J, et al. Epidemiology of severe sepsis in the United States: analysis of incidence, outcome, and associated costs of care. Crit Care Med 2001. https://doi.org/10.1097/00003246-200107000-00002.

36. Rhodes A, Evans LE, Alhazzani W, et al. Surviving sepsis campaign: international guidelines for management of sepsis and septic shock: 2016. Crit Care Med 2017. https://doi.org/10.1097/CCM.0000000000002255.

37. Woznica EA, Inglot M, Woznica RK, et al. Liver dysfunction in sepsis. Adv Clin Exp Med 2018. https://doi.org/10.17219/acem/68363.

38. Brierre S, Kumari R, Deboisblanc BP. The endocrine system during sepsis. Am J Med Sci 2004. https://doi.org/10.1097/00000441-200410000-00007.

39. Marik PE, Zaloga GP. Adrenal insufficiency during septic shock. Crit Care Med 2003. https://doi.org/10.1097/00003246-200301000-00022.

40. Sharshar T, Blanchard A, Paillard M, et al. Circulating vasopressin levels in septic shock. Crit Care Med 2003. https://doi.org/10.1097/01.CCM.0000063046.82359.4A.

41. Chopra IJ. Euthyroid sick syndrome: is it a misnomer? J Clin Endocrinol Metab 1997. https://doi.org/10.1210/jcem.82.2.3745.

42. Sonneville R, Verdonk F, Rauturier C, et al. Understanding brain dysfunction in sepsis. Ann Intensive Care 2013. https://doi.org/10.1186/2110-5820-3-15.

43. Rivers E, Nguyen B, Havstad S, et al. Early goal-directed therapy in the treatment of severe sepsis and septic shock. N Engl J Med 2001;345(19):1368–77.

44. Yealy D, Kellum J, Huang D, et al. A randomized trial of protocol-based care for early septic shock. N Engl J Med 2014;47(2):256–7.

45. Peake SL, Bailey M, Bellomo R, et al. Australasian Resuscitation of Sepsis Evaluation (ARISE): a multi-centre, prospective, inception cohort study. Resuscitation 2009;80(7):811–8.

46. Mouncey PR, Osborn TM, Power GS, et al. Trial of early, goal-directed resuscitation for septic shock. N Engl J Med 2015;372(14):1301–11.

47. Pepper DJ, Sun J, Rhee C, et al. Procalcitonin-guided antibiotic discontinuation and mortality in critically ill adults: a systematic review and meta-analysis. Chest 2019;155(6):1109–18.

48. Levy MM, Evans LE, Rhodes A. The surviving sepsis campaign bundle: 2018 update. Crit Care Med 2018;46:997–1000.

49. Singer M. Antibiotics for sepsis: does each hour really count, or is it incestuous amplification? Am J Respir Crit Care Med 2017;196(7):800–2.

50. Kumar A, Roberts D, Wood KE, et al. Duration of hypotension before initiation of effective antimicrobial therapy is the critical determinant of survival in human septic shock. Crit Care Med 2006;34(6):1589–96.

51. Acheampong A, Vincent J-L. A positive fluid balance is an independent prognostic factor in patients with sepsis. Crit Care 2015;19(1). https://doi.org/10.1186/s13054-015-0970-1.

52. Muller L, Toumi M, Bousquet P-J, et al. An increase in aortic blood flow after an infusion of 100 ml colloid over 1 minute can predict fluid responsiveness. Anesthesiology 2011;115(3):541–7.

53. Wu Y, Zhou S, Zhou Z, et al. A 10-second fluid challenge guided by transthoracic echocardiography can predict fluid responsiveness. Crit Care 2014;18(3):1–8.

54. Muller L, Bobbia X, Toumi M, et al. Respiratory variations of inferior vena cava diameter to predict fluid responsiveness in spontaneously breathing patients with acute circulatory failure: need for a cautious use. Crit Care 2012;16(5):R188.

55. Marik PE, Cavallazzi R, Vasu T, et al. Dynamic changes in arterial waveform derived variables and fluid responsiveness in mechanically ventilated patients: a systematic review of the literature. Crit Care Med 2009;37(9):2642–7.

56. Maheshwari K, Nathanson BH, Munson SH, et al. The relationship between ICU hypotension and in-hospital mortality and morbidity in septic patients. Intensive Care Med 2018;44(6):857–67.

57. Khanna AK, Maheshwari K, Mao G, et al. Association between mean arterial pressure and acute kidney injury and a composite of myocardial injury and mortality in postoperative critically ill patients: a retrospective cohort analysis. Crit Care Med 2019. https://doi.org/10.1097/CCM.0000000000003763.

58. Asfar P, Meziani F, Hamel JF, et al. High versus low blood-pressure target in patients with septic shock. N Engl J Med 2014;370(17):1583–93.

59. Khanna AK. Defending a mean arterial pressure in the intensive care unit: are we there yet? Ann Intensive Care 2018;8(1):4–5.

60. Asfar P, Radermacher P, Ostermann M. MAP of 65: target of the past? Intensive Care Med 2018;44(9):1551–2.

61. De Backer DP, Biston P, Devriendt J, et al. Comparison of dopamine and norepinephrine in the treatment of shock. N Engl J Med 2010;362(9):1543–54.

62. Dellinger RP, Mitchell M, Levy, et al. Surviving sepsis campaign: international guidelines for management of severe sepsis and septic shock, 2012. Intensive Care Med 2013;39(2):165–228.

63. Myburgh JA, Higgins A, Jovanovska A, et al. A comparison of epinephrine and norepinephrine in critically ill patients. Intensive Care Med 2008;34(12):2226–34.
64. Avni T, Lador A, Lev S, et al. Vasopressors for the treatment of septic shock: systematic review and meta-analysis. PLoS One 2015. https://doi.org/10.1371/journal.pone.0129305.
65. Russell J, Walley K, Singer J, et al. Vasopressin versus norepinephrine infusion in patients with septic shock. N Engl J Med 2008;358(9):877–87.
66. Khanna A, English SW, Wang XS, et al. Angiotensin II for the treatment of vasodilatory shock. N Engl J Med 2017;377(5):419–30.
67. Brown SM, Lanspa MJ, Jones JP, et al. Survival after shock requiring high-dose vasopressor therapy. Chest 2013. https://doi.org/10.1378/chest.12-1106.
68. Venkatesh B, Khanna AK, Cohen J. Less is more: catecholamine-sparing strategies in septic shock. Intensive Care Med 2019;14–6. https://doi.org/10.1007/s00134-019-05770-3.
69. Venkatesh B, Finfer S, Cohen J, et al. Adjunctive glucocorticoid therapy in patients with septic shock. N Engl J Med 2018;378(9):797–808.
70. Annane D, Renault A, Brun-Buisson C, et al. Hydrocortisone plus fludrocortisone for adults with septic shock. N Engl J Med 2018;378(9):809–18.
71. Marik PE, Khangoora V, Rivera R, et al. Hydrocortisone, vitamin C, and thiamine for the treatment of severe sepsis and septic shock: a retrospective before-after study. Chest 2017;151(6):1229–38.
72. Zabet M, Mohammadi M, Ramezani M, et al. Effect of high-dose ascorbic acid on vasopressor's requirement in septic shock. J Res Pharm Pract 2016;5(2):94.
73. Fowler AA, Truwit JD, Hite RD, et al. Effect of vitamin C infusion on organ failure and biomarkers of inflammation and vascular injury in patients with sepsis and severe acute respiratory failure: the CITRIS-ALI randomized clinical trial. JAMA 2019;322(13):1261–70.

Management of Pneumonia Syndromes in the Hospital: Make Pneumonia Your Best Friend

Abraham Kanal, MD, Bradley A. Sharpe, MD*, Jesse Abelson, MD

KEYWORDS

- Pneumonia • Community-acquired pneumonia • Hospital-acquired pneumonia
- Ventilator-associated pneumonia • Aspiration pneumonia • Antibiotics

KEY POINTS

- Viruses may cause CAP more commonly than previously recognized, although the causative organism is rarely identified.
- The diagnosis of CAP remains clinical. Given the limitations of CXR, point-of-care ultrasound and chest CT scanning can be used as adjuncts.
- In the treatment of CAP in the hospital, risk factors for MRSA and *Pseudomonas aeruginosa* can help guide empiric therapy; these include patients with either prior isolation of the organism or receipt of parenteral antibiotics in the prior 90 days.
- Most patients hospitalized with CAP should receive 5 days of antibiotic therapy; those with HAP or VAP should receive 7 days of therapy.
- Treatment of HAP and VAP should generally include coverage of MRSA and resistant gram-negative organisms.

Pneumonia may well be called the friend of the aged. Taken off by it in an acute, not often painful illness, the old man escapes those "cold gradations of decay" so distressing to himself and his friends.

—William Osler, 1898

INTRODUCTION

Pneumonia syndromes are defined as acute infections of the pulmonary parenchyma. The most common pneumonia syndromes in the hospital include:

- Community-acquired pneumonia (CAP): acquired outside of the hospital setting

Division of Hospital Medicine, Department of Medicine, University of California San Francisco (UCSF), Box 0131, San Francisco, CA 94143, USA
* Corresponding author.
E-mail address: Bradley.Sharpe@ucsf.edu
Twitter: @AbelsonJesse (J.A.)

Med Clin N Am 104 (2020) 587–599
https://doi.org/10.1016/j.mcna.2020.02.006
0025-7125/20/© 2020 Elsevier Inc. All rights reserved.

medical.theclinics.com

- Hospital-acquired pneumonia (HAP): acquired ≥ 48 hours after admission to the hospital
- Ventilator-associated pneumonia (VAP): acquired ≥ 48 hours after endotracheal intubation
- Aspiration pneumonia: acquired outside or inside the hospital setting after inhalation of gastric contents

Pneumonia syndromes cause significant morbidity and mortality. This article provides a comprehensive review of the common syndromes with a particular focus on CAP.

COMMUNITY-ACQUIRED PNEUMONIA
Microbiology

The understanding of the microbiology of CAP has evolved in recent years. Classic teaching held that most CAP was caused by typical bacteria (eg, *Streptococcus pneumoniae*) with some contribution from atypical bacteria (eg, *Mycoplasma* spp). Recent evidence suggests the microbiology may be more complex with increasing contributions from respiratory viruses.

A large study evaluated patients admitted to the hospital with CAP with a broad array of diagnostic tests including blood and sputum cultures, urine antigen testing, and any available polymerase chain reaction testing.[1] The authors failed to detect a pathogen in 62% of patients. The following pathogens were identified:

- A virus (23%)
- A bacteria (11%)
- Both (3%)

Rhinovirus (9%), influenza (6%), and *S pneumoniae* (5%) were the most frequently identified. Atypical pathogens were identified in only 4%. The authors posited few sputum specimens and the adoption of the childhood pneumococcal vaccine as reasons for the low overall yield and the low rate of *S pneumoniae*, respectively.

In an alternative study, molecular testing resulted in pathogen detection in 87% of patients, which included bacteria in 81%, virus in 30%, and coinfection with both in 24%. Common CAP bacterial pathogens predominated (eg, *S pneumoniae*).[2]

As diagnostic testing improves, the understanding of the microbiology will evolve. The evidence does suggest viruses play a prominent role but the usual bacterial organisms are still commonly present.

Concern has been raised about the rising prevalence of community-acquired methicillin-resistant *Staphylococcus aureus* (MRSA) as a cause of severe CAP. Studies have revealed community-acquired MRSA is actually uncommon; it may be the causative agent in less than 3% of cases.[3] Certain risk factors can increase the likelihood of MRSA (**Box 1**) and these risk factors need to be considered when deciding on appropriate empiric therapy.

Box 1
Risk factors for infection from MRSA or *Pseudomonas aeruginosa*

Patients with either of the following:
- Prior respiratory isolation of the organism
- Received parenteral antibiotics within the prior 90 days

Data from Metlay JP, Waterer GW, Long AC, et al. Diagnosis and treatment of adults with community-acquired pneumonia. An official clinical practice guideline of the American Thoracic Society and Infectious Diseases Society of America. Am J Respir Crit Care Med 2019;200(7):e45-67.

In real-world settings, the causative organism is not identified in most patients with CAP.[4] Given the limitations of the standard diagnostic tests, empirical therapy must target typical and atypical organisms and, when relevant, influenza infection.

Lastly, the fundamental understanding of the microbiology of the lungs is changing. The pulmonary parenchyma has long been presumed to be a sterile space. Yet, recent work suggests CAP may be increasingly understood as a dysbiosis (an imbalance in the types of organism present in an individual's natural microflora).[4] The implications of such an understanding are difficult to predict but could fundamentally change how one thinks about the treatment of CAP.

Diagnosis

The diagnosis of pneumonia remains clinical, based on a combination of:[5]

- Signs or symptoms of pneumonia (which can include fever, confusion, new or worsening cough, sputum production, dyspnea, etc.) and
- Evidence of new pulmonary infiltrate on imaging

Unfortunately, there are no historical features or examination signs that are accurate enough to make the diagnosis of CAP without imaging.[6]

Imaging

The 2019 Infectious Diseases Society of America (IDSA)/American Thoracic Society (ATS) CAP guidelines emphasize that the diagnosis of pneumonia has a radiographic component but do not comment on a preference for a particular imaging modality[7]

The chest radiograph (CXR) remains the most frequently used diagnostic test but has limitations. A 2012 study enrolled 3423 patients who presented to the emergency department with at least one of shortness of breath, chest pain, or cough. All patients received CXR and chest computed tomography (CT). They found that CXR was 43.5% sensitive and 93% specific for pulmonary opacity.[8] In a smaller 2015 study that evaluated patients specifically suspected of CAP who received a chest CT within 4 hours, CXR performed poorly. CT scans revealed an infiltrate in 33% of patients with no infiltrate on CXR and excluded CAP in 30% of patients with an infiltrate on CXR.[9] In a patient with consistent symptoms, a clear infiltrate on CXR likely does indicate pneumonia but absence does not reliably rule out the diagnosis.

Point-of-care ultrasound is an increasingly used modality to diagnose CAP. When chest CT is used as a reference, bedside ultrasound has a sensitivity of 85% to 95% and a specificity of 75% to 90%.[10] Overall performance is believed to be better than CXR.[10] An important limitation is the need for provider expertise in the acquisition and interpretation of images. As the technology and skill become more ubiquitous, point-of-care ultrasound may become an important modality in the diagnosis of CAP.

Chest CT is usually used as the reference standard to delineate pulmonary infiltrates. That said, it is not always clear when to order a CT scan and the decision to do so is highly provider dependent. We recommend chest CT when there is one of the following:

- High clinical suspicion of pneumonia but a negative CXR
- Suspicion of a false-positive CXR
- Suspicion of an alternative diagnosis (eg, pulmonary embolism)
- To evaluate for potential causes of treatment failure (eg, abscess or empyema)

Patterns of CT use may change in the next decade as protocols with less radiation exposure and lower cost become available.[4]

Procalcitonin

There is increasing interest that procalcitonin can be used in CAP (and other diseases) to help differentiate bacterial infections from other infections. Multiple studies have shown that procalcitonin is elevated in bacterial infections and low or normal in viral or other infections.[11] Hope has persisted that procalcitonin might discriminate a population of patients with pneumonia who are unlikely to have a bacterial cause and so can reasonably be spared antibiotic therapy. A decrease in procalcitonin level has also been studied to identify patients for whom antibiotics might be stopped early.

Although procalcitonin has demonstrated promise, the 2019 IDSA/ATS CAP guidelines recommend against its use in patients who are believed to have CAP.[7] This is based on several key factors:

- Poor at ruling out atypical bacterial infections and mixed bacterial and viral infections
- Inability to adequately rule out bacterial infection at the time of presentation (antibiotics must be initiated if the patient has clinical pneumonia)
- Unlikely to reduce antibiotic exposure if used to decide about stopping antibiotics given recommendations for shorter courses of antibiotics (discussed in Treatment section)

Other Studies

In most patients hospitalized for CAP, the causative organism cannot be identified even with appropriate diagnostic testing.[4] The 2019 IDSA/ATS CAP guidelines strongly recommend attempts to identify a causative organism in two cohorts of patients[7]:

- Those with risk factors for MRSA and/or *Pseudomonas aeruginosa* (see **Box 1**)
- Patients with severe CAP (**Box 2**)

In these patients, blood and sputum cultures are recommended. Note, in other patients hospitalized with CAP who do not meet these criteria, blood and sputum cultures should not routinely be ordered. They are unlikely to yield an organism and

---

Box 2
Criteria for defining severe community-acquired pneumonia

Definition includes either 1 major criteria or 3 or more minor criteria

Minor criteria
- Respiratory rate greater than 30 breaths/min
- Pao_2/Fio_2 ratio less than 250
- Multilobar infiltrates
- Confusion/disorientation
- Uremia
- Leukopenia
- Thrombocytopenia
- Hypothermia
- Hypotension requiring intravenous fluids

Major criteria
- Septic shock with need for vasopressors
- Respiratory failure requiring ventilation

Adapted from Mandell LA, Wunderink RG, Anzueto A, et. al. Infectious Diseases Society of America/American Thoracic Society Consensus Guidelines on the Management of Community-Acquired Pneumonia in Adults. Clin Infect Dis 2007;44(Suppl 2):S38.

the risk of identifying organisms because of contamination (and confusion) is high.[7] The guidelines also recommend not routinely sending urine pneumococcal antigen or urine *Legionella* antigen as there are flaws with the test characteristics and utility of both tests.[7]

Treatment

Treatment overview

Despite advances in the understanding of the microbiology of CAP, there remain significant challenges in real-world settings in identifying causative agents and patients at increased risk for antibiotic-resistant pathogens. As such, treatment remains largely empiric. Prior guidelines and the overly inclusive category of health care–associated pneumonia (HCAP) led to vast overuse of unnecessarily broad-spectrum antibiotics in the past decade without evidence of improved outcomes.[12]

A concerted effort toward antibiotic stewardship motivated the 2019 ATS/IDSA update to suggest multiple changes as follows[7]:

- Doing away with HCAP classification
- A preference for shorter courses of antibiotics
- Avoiding anaerobic coverage for aspiration
- Choosing broad-spectrum coverage based on local and individualized epidemiologic data and validated severity indices

General treatment strategies

Established sepsis guidelines and large, multicenter studies of patients with CAP suggest benefit from a standardized approach (eg, care bundles) to CAP treatment. These bundles can include rapid and adequate fluid resuscitation, risk stratification, early measurement and correction of hypoxia, early ambulation, and maintenance of electrolyte and glucose homeostasis.[13] Institutions are encouraged to develop such bundles and incorporate them into the electronic medical record.

Antibiotics and treatment hierarchy

Selection of an antibiotic regimen in CAP continues to be guided by location (outpatient, inpatient, intensive care unit [ICU]), comorbidities, risk factors for resistant organisms, and disease severity.[7] The guideline-recommended antibiotic regimens for outpatients with CAP are beyond the scope of this review but are found in the IDSA/ATS guidelines.[7]

Treatment of inpatient community-acquired pneumonia

For inpatients, empiric regimens are guided by severity of illness and risk factors for resistant organisms. The most recent guidelines suggest using previously described criteria for severe CAP (see **Box 2**).[5,7] Although we agree with these criteria, in practical management, "severe CAP" is more easily defined by the presence of any of the following:

- Septic shock
- Respiratory failure requiring mechanical ventilation
- Other factors requiring ICU admission

Nonsevere community-acquired pneumonia

For nonsevere CAP (ie, non-ICU), the single most optimal regimen remains unclear despite large, multicenter trials and subsequent meta-analyses. Overall, the evidence supports antibiotic selection that empirically treats traditional typical and atypical organisms.[14]

The guidelines suggest three potential regimens to treat nonsevere CAP (**Box 3**)[7]:

- Combination β-lactam (eg, ceftriaxone) plus macrolide (eg, azithromycin)
- Monotherapy with a respiratory fluoroquinolone (eg, levofloxacin)
- Combination β-lactam plus doxycycline (most useful for patients with both macrolide and fluoroquinolone intolerance)

In selecting one regimen over others, hospital-based providers should consider using local antibiograms and prescribing patterns. Of note, a recent study suggests doxycycline may have a lower incidence of *Clostridium difficile* infection in the setting of CAP requiring hospitalization.[15] Doxycycline may also have lower out-of-pocket costs for patients.

Severe community-acquired pneumonia

In general for severe CAP, the microbiology is the same as nonsevere CAP. Yet, patients with severe pneumonia are most likely to have resistant organisms and broader coverage can be considered. Combination therapy is standard. Guidelines-recommended regimens include[7]

- A β-lactam plus a macrolide or
- A β-lactam plus a respiratory fluoroquinolone

We prefer a β-lactam plus a macrolide because a meta-analysis of observational data favors macrolide-containing regimens based on a potential mortality benefit when compared with other regimens.[16] The ATS/IDSA guidelines suggest including a macrolide when treating severe CAP and caution against fluoroquinolone monotherapy or combination β-lactam/doxycycline.[7] All patients with severe CAP should have blood and sputum cultures. Empiric treatment of MRSA (eg, vancomycin) and *P aeruginosa* (eg, piperacillin/tazobactam) is not necessary for all patients with severe CAP. This decision should be reserved for patients with specific risk factors (see **Box 2**).

Response to treatment

Typically, significant clinical response is expected within 24 to 48 hours after initiation of antibiotic therapy.[17] Clinical worsening or slow/absent response should quickly raise suspicion for a resistant organism, an atypical organism, a complication of pneumonia (eg, empyema), or an alternative diagnosis (eg, interstitial lung disease). Moreover, symptoms can persist; in one study of the natural history of CAP, nearly 90% of patients had at least one pneumonia-related symptom (eg, cough, shortness of breath, chest pain) at 30 days.[18] This information is important when counseling patients at the time of discharge.

Duration of therapy

A growing body of evidence continues to suggest noninferiority of shorter regimens compared with longer regimens. A randomized controlled trial in 2016 showed that in hospitalized patients with nonsevere CAP who had clinically improved and were afebrile after 48 hours, treatment with 5 days had similar mortality and clinical response to a longer course (approximately 10 days).[19] Based on this and other prior studies, the new 2019 IDSA/ATS CAP guidelines recommend treatment for 5 days for most patients.[7] One caveat is patients must be clinically improved and afebrile. Some patients with CAP are slower to respond and may need 7 days of therapy. Nearly 30% of patients in the previously mentioned randomized controlled trial received more than 5 days based on the discretion of the provider.[19] Extension to 7 days should also be considered for those with suspected or proven MRSA or pseudomonal CAP.[7] De-escalation to regimens with narrower antimicrobial spectra is guided by any available microbiologic data.

For future directions, initial studies have shown promise for the antimicrobials omadacycline (a tetracycline) and lefamulin (a novel pleuromutilin antibiotic) for CAP, although high cost and sparse safety data limit their current utility.

Adjunctive Treatments

Corticosteroids

In patients with CAP, some of the lung injury that can lead to respiratory failure is not from the causative organism but rather from the host's inflammatory response. With this understanding, multiple studies investigating the utility of systemic corticosteroids in CAP have been performed, leading to several large meta-analyses and systematic reviews.[20–23] Overall, these collectively suggest a possible reduction in length of stay, antibiotic duration, and perhaps even mortality with an increase in hyperglycemia. Yet the data are heterogeneous and of only low-to-moderate quality. Based on this, the most recent ATS CAP guidelines recommend against routinely using corticosteroids in the treatment of CAP.[7]

Given the overall data and a potential for real clinical and survival benefits, the authors believe it is reasonable to consider using adjunctive steroids for patients with severe CAP. Specific steroid, dose, and duration varied across the major studies but based on the largest study, a proposed regimen is prednisone 50 mg/d (or equivalent in methylprednisolone) for 7 days.[20]

Antiviral therapy

Viruses are often discovered in patients presenting with CAP. Yet, the pathogenicity of these viruses and the possibility of coinfection with bacteria make interpretation of these results challenging. It is not clear that if a virus (eg, respiratory syncytial virus) is identified in a patient with CAP, it is safe to stop empiric antibacterial therapy. In the hospital setting, given morbidity and mortality associated with not treating bacterial pneumonia, it is typically appropriate to continue the antibacterial treatment in this situation.

During influenza season, empiric oseltamivir should be initiated in patients presenting with CAP. In patients with identified influenza pneumonia, treatment with oseltamivir likely leads to more rapid clinical improvement and lower mortality.[24] The ATS/IDSA guidelines suggest there may be a role for premature cessation of antibiotic therapy in patients with CAP and confirmed influenza who improve rapidly after initiation of antiviral therapy.[7] This decision can be made at the providers discretion based on the clinical circumstances.

Miscellaneous

Cardiovascular disease

The observational relationship between hospitalization for CAP and subsequent cardiovascular disease has been well-established. The association includes an increased risk for myocardial infarction, stroke, and fatal coronary heart disease.[25,26] A growing body of retrospective research has begun to explore whether concomitant antiplatelet or statin therapy might offer benefit in reducing the incidence of these comorbid outcomes.[27,28] Prospective studies are needed to further investigate this high-risk area of overlap and to determine whether there is a role to initiate these agents de novo for patients hospitalized with CAP.

HEALTH CARE–ASSOCIATED PNEUMONIA

ATS guidelines published in 2005 defined a new category of pneumonia: HCAP.[29] Research had revealed higher prevalence of resistant organisms in patients with health care exposure.[30] In the guideline, patients were classified as having HCAP if they had one of the following: hospitalization in the previous 90 days, residence in a nursing facility, hemodialysis, or receipt of homecare (eg, antibiotics, wound care). Since the publication of these guidelines, extensive evidence has revealed these criteria do not accurately predict antibiotic-resistant pathogens and this classification has led to excessive use of broad-spectrum antibiotics with no impact on outcomes.[12,31] Because of this, HCAP was not included in the most recent HAP/VAP guidelines and is no longer viewed as a valid classification of pneumonia type.[32] Instead, in a patient with CAP, the decision about coverage of resistant organisms (eg, MRSA, P aeruginosa) should be based on the individual risk factors that are strongly predictive (see **Box 1**) and local microbiology (eg, high prevalence of MRSA causing CAP requiring ICU admission).

HOSPITAL-ACQUIRED PNEUMONIA AND VENTILATOR-ASSOCIATED PNEUMONIA

HAP and VAP are associated with morbidity, resource use, and mortality.[33] HAP is defined as "pneumonia not incubating at the time of admission, and occurring greater than 48 hours from admission," whereas VAP is similarly defined as "pneumonia occurring greater than 48 hours after endotracheal intubation."[32]

Microbiology and Diagnosis

Prevalent pathogens in HAP and VAP differ considerably from those in routine CAP and include: S aureus (methicillin-sensitive and methicillin-resistant), P aeruginosa, and other enteric gram-negative bacilli. S pneumoniae, a dominant pathogen in CAP, may contribute to HAP outside the ICU.[34]

The gold standard for diagnosis of HAP and VAP remains elusive. In general, clinical and radiographic evidence of pneumonia should lead the clinician to obtain noninvasive microbiologic tests of disease. These include blood cultures and sampling of respiratory secretions, whether from produced or induced sputum in HAP or nasotracheal/endotracheal aspiration in VAP (or HAP patients who are subsequently ventilated).

Treatment

As in CAP, treatment of HAP or VAP begins with careful risk stratification. Recent guidelines encourage clinicians to incorporate the following to determine the need for empiric therapy against multidrug-resistant organisms (MDRO)[32]:

- Regional, institutional, and unit-based antibiogram data
- Individual risk factors, prior culture data, and disease severity

Empiric therapy for HAP and VAP should generally include coverage for *S aureus* and for gram-negative rods. Selection of specific antibiotic regimens depends on risk factors for MRSA and risk factors for drug-resistant gram-negatives. Risk factors for MRSA in the setting of HAP and VAP include[32]

- Treatment in a unit where greater than 10%–20% of *S aureus* isolates are methicillin-resistant
- Treatment in a unit where the prevalence of MRSA is not known
- Colonization with MRSA or prior isolation of MRSA

Risk factors for multidrug-resistant gram-negative organisms in the hospital include[32]

- Intravenous antibiotic use within the previous 90 days
- Septic shock at the time of HAP/VAP
- Acute respiratory distress syndrome preceding HAP/VAP
- ≥5 days of hospitalization before the occurrence of HAP/VAP
- Acute renal-replacement therapy before HAP/VAP onset

Patients with HAP or VAP without MRSA or MDRO risk factors can generally be treated with monotherapy including: piperacillin-tazobactam, cefepime, imipenem, or meropenem. If patients have MRSA risk factors, then vancomycin or linezolid should be added.[32]

If a patient with HAP or VAP is critically ill or has MDRO risk factors, clinicians should consider treating with two gram-negative agents. Providers can choose from two of the following: piperacillin-tazobactam, cefepime, levofloxacin, imipenem or meropenem, tobramycin, or aztreonam.[32]

De-escalation

The recent guidelines emphasize prompt species identification and early transition to narrowed, tailored regimens when possible.[32] Yet, similar to CAP, often the causative organism cannot be identified in patients with HAP or VAP. Under these circumstances, if a patient is clinically improving, in general the antibiotics should be de-escalated, that is, changed to a more narrow-spectrum antibiotic or to monotherapy if treated with multiple agents.

A recent retrospective study showed shorter length of stay, lower acute kidney injury, and no difference in mortality when patients with HAP or VAP without an identified organism had *S aureus* coverage discontinued by Day 4.[35] In patients with HAP or VAP with unknown microbiology who are clinically improving, in general providers should stop the *S aureus* coverage on Day 3 and can often transition to an oral fluoroquinolone shortly thereafter.

Duration of Therapy

A typical regimen for either HAP or VAP should be for at least 7 days, although regimens may be reasonably abridged (rarely to fewer than 5 days) or extended based on provider discretion.[32,36] Neither procalcitonin nor clinical pulmonary infection score are recommended to guide initiation or duration of therapy.[32]

ASPIRATION

Aspiration of small amounts of oropharyngeal contents is common; in one study, 45% of healthy adults had some aspiration while sleeping.[37] In patients with depressed consciousness, dysphagia, or other risk factors, aspiration of larger amounts of material can lead to several aspiration syndromes:

- Aspiration pneumonitis
- Aspiration pneumonia
- Pulmonary abscess

When gastric contents (eg, vomit, undigested food, liquids) are aspirated, the initial response is a chemical pneumonitis, a noninfectious inflammatory response.[38] Pneumonitis can present with fever, cough, wheezing, or hypoxia, and in rare cases can lead to acute respiratory distress syndrome.[39] Patients typically recover over the course of hours and typically do not need antibiotic therapy.

True aspiration pneumonia typically develops 48 to 72 hours after the aspiration event, which represents the time necessary for bacterial replication, and can present with respiratory symptoms or nonrespiratory symptoms in the elderly (eg, confusion, falls).[40] It was a long-standing belief that anaerobes were the main organism involved in true aspiration pneumonia. Studies have revealed this is not the case and that, for most patients with true aspiration pneumonia, the microbiology is similar to the microbiology of CAP or HAP.[38,39] Although there is not clear evidence, most patients with true aspiration pneumonia can be treated similar to patients with CAP and HAP (discussed in Treatment and HAP/VAP sections).

Pulmonary abscess is a unique clinical scenario where the presentation is more indolent; patients typically present weeks to a month after the aspiration events. Symptoms typically include low-grade fever, cough with purulent sputum, and general malaise. Pulmonary abscesses are often polymicrobial, including anaerobes. Therefore, therapy should include anaerobic coverage; a β-lactam with a β-lactam inhibitor is appropriate.

SUMMARY

Pneumonia syndromes are common in hospital medicine and lead to substantial morbidity and mortality. The evidence and guidelines provide clear recommendations on management strategies. Future research will provide more insight into the microbiology, optimal diagnostic testing, and best therapeutic options for these syndromes.

DISCLOSURE

The authors have nothing to disclose.

REFERENCES

1. Jain S, Self WH, Wunderink RG, et al, CDC EPIC Study Team. Community-acquired pneumonia requiring hospitalization among U.S. adults. N Engl J Med 2015;373:415–27.

2. Gadsby NJ, Russell CD, McHugh MP, et al. Comprehensive molecular testing for respiratory pathogens in community-acquired pneumonia. Clin Infect Dis 2016; 62(7):817–23.

3. Self WH, Wunderlink RG, Williams DJ, et al. *Staphylococcus aureus* community-acquired pneumonia: prevalence, clinical characteristics, and outcomes. Clin Infect Dis 2016;63(3):300–9.

4. Wunderink R, Waterer G. Advances in the causes and management of community acquired pneumonia in adults. BMJ 2017;358:2471–84.

5. Mandell LA, Wunderlink RG, Anzueto A, et al. Infectious Diseases Society of America/American Thoracic Society consensus guidelines on the management of community-acquired pneumonia in adults. Clin Infect Dis 2007;44(Suppl 2): S27–72.

6. Metlay JP, Kapoor WN, Fine MJ. Does this patient have community-acquired pneumonia? Diagnosing pneumonia by history and physical examination. JAMA 1997;278:1440–5.

7. Metlay JP, Waterer GW, Long AC, et al. Diagnosis and treatment of adults with community-acquired pneumonia. An official practice guideline of the American Thoracic Society and Infectious Diseases Society of America. Am J Respir Crit Care Med 2019;200:e45–67.

8. Self WH, Courtney DM, McNaughton CD, et al. High discordance of chest x-ray and computed tomography for detection of pulmonary opacities in ED patients: implications for diagnosing pneumonia. Am J Emerg Med 2013;31:401–5.

9. Claessens YE, Deborah MP, Tubach F, et al. Early chest computed tomography scan to assist diagnosis and guide treatment decision for suspected community-acquired pneumonia. Am J Respir Crit Care Med 2015;192:974–82.

10. Staub LJ, Mazzali Biscaro RR, Kaszubowski E, et al. Lung ultrasound for the emergency diagnosis of pneumonia, acute heart failure, and exacerbations of chronic obstructive pulmonary disease/asthma in adults: a systematic review and meta-analysis. J Emerg Med 2019;56:53–69.

11. Gilbert DN. Use of plasma procalcitonin levels as an adjunct to clinical microbiology. J Clin Microbiol 2010;48(7):2325.

12. Rothberg MB, Zilberberg MD, Pekow PS, et al. Association of guideline-based antimicrobial therapy and outcomes in healthcare-associated pneumonia. J Antimicrob Chemother 2015;70:1573–9.

13. Lim WS, Rodrigo C, Turner AM, et al. British Thoracic Society community-acquired pneumonia care bundle: results of a national implementation project. Thorax 2016;71:288–90.

14. Lee JS, Giesler DL, Gellad WF, et al. Antibiotic therapy for adults hospitalized with community-acquired pneumonia: a systematic review. JAMA 2016;315:593–602.

15. Doernberg SB, Winston LG, Deck DH, et al. Does doxycycline protect against development of *Clostridium difficile* infection? Clin Infect Dis 2012;55(5):615–20.

16. Sligl WI, Asadi L, Eurich DT, et al. Macrolides and mortality in critically ill patients with community-acquired pneumonia: a systematic review and meta-analysis. Crit Care Med 2014;42(2):420–32.

17. Halm EA, Fine MJ, Marrie TJ, et al. Time to clinical stability in patients hospitalized with community-acquired pneumonia: implications for practice guidelines. JAMA 1998;279:1452.

18. Fine MJ, Stone RA, Singer DE, et al. Processes and outcomes of care for patients with community-acquired pneumonia: results from the Pneumonia Patient Outcomes Research Team (PORT) cohort study. Arch Intern Med 1999;159:970.

19. Uranga A, Espana PP, Bilbao A, et al. Duration of antibiotic treatment in community-acquired pneumonia: a multicenter randomized clinical trial. JAMA Intern Med 2016;176(9):1257–65.

20. Huang J, Guo J, Li H, et al. Efficacy and safety of adjunctive corticosteroids therapy for patients with severe community-acquired pneumonia: a systematic review and meta-analysis. Medicine (Baltimore) 2019;98:13–21.

21. Briel M, Spoorenberg SMC, Snijders D, et al. Corticosteroids in patients hospitalized with community-acquired pneumonia: systematic review and individual patient data metaanalysis. Clin Infect Dis 2018;66(3):346–54.

22. Wan Y, Sun T, Liu Z, et al. Efficacy and safety of corticosteroids for community-acquired pneumonia: a systematic review and meta-analysis. Chest 2016; 149(1):209–19.

23. Siemieniuk RAC, Meade MO, Alonso-Coella P, et al. Corticosteroid therapy for patients hospitalized with community-acquired pneumonia: a systematic review and meta-analysis. Ann Intern Med 2015;163:519–28.

24. Doll MK, Winters N, Boikos C, et al. Safety and effectiveness of neuraminidase inhibitors for influenza treatment, prophylaxis, and outbreak control: a systematic review of systematic reviews and/or meta-analyses. J Antimicrob Chemother 2017;72(11):2990–3007.

25. Corrales-Medina VF, Alvarez KN, Weissfeld LA, et al. Association between hospitalization for pneumonia and subsequent risk of cardiovascular disease. JAMA 2015;313(3):264–74.

26. Kwong JC, Schwartz KL, Campitelli MA, et al. Acute myocardial infarction after laboratory-confirmed influenza infection. N Engl J Med 2018;378:345–53.

27. Gross AK, Dunn SP, Feola DJ, et al. Clopidogrel treatment on the incidence and severity of community acquired pneumonia in a cohort study and metaanalysis of antiplatelet therapy in pneumonia and critical illness. J Thromb Thrombolysis 2013;35(2):147–54.

28. Chalmers JD, Singanayagam A, Murray MP, et al. Prior statin use is associated with improved outcomes in community-acquired pneumonia. Am J Med 2008; 121(11):1002–7.

29. American Thoracic Society, Infectious Diseases Society of America. Guidelines for the management of adults with hospital-acquired, ventilator-associated, and healthcare-associated pneumonia. Am J Respir Crit Care Med 2005;17(4): 388–416.

30. Kollef MH, Shorr A, Tabak YP, et al. Epidemiology and outcomes of health-care-associated pneumonia: results from a large US database of culture-positive pneumonia. Chest 2005;128(6):3854–62.

31. Chalmers JD, Rother C, Salih W, et al. Healthcare-associated pneumonia does not accurately identify potentially resistant pathogens: a systematic review and meta-analysis. Clin Infect Dis 2014;58:330–9.

32. Kalil AC, Metersky ML, Klompas M, et al. Management of adults with hospital-acquired and ventilator-associated pneumonia: 2016 clinical practice guidelines by the Infectious Diseases Society of America and the American Thoracic Society. Clin Infect Dis 2016;63(5):e61–111.

33. Muscedere JG, Day A, Heyland DK. Mortality, attributable mortality, and clinical events as end points for clinical trials of ventilator-associated pneumonia and hospital-acquired pneumonia. Clin Infect Dis 2010;51(suppl 1): S120–5.

34. Sopena N, Sabria M, Neunos 2000 Study Group. Multicenter study of hospital-acquired pneumonia in non-ICU patients. Chest 2005;127(1):213–9.

35. Cowley MC, Ritchie DJ, Hampton N, et al. Outcomes associated with de-escalating therapy for methicillin-resistant Staphylococcus aureus in culture-negative nosocomial pneumonia. Chest 2019;155(1):53–9.

36. Dimopoulos G, Poulakaou G, Pneumatikos IA, et al. Short- vs. long-duration antibiotic regiments for ventilator-associated pneumonia: a systematic review and meta-analysis. Chest 2013;144(6):1759–67.

37. Huxley EJ, Viroslav J, Gray WR, et al. Pharyngeal aspiration in normal adults and patients with depressed consciousness. Am J Med 1978;64(4):564–8.

38. Marik PE. Aspiration pneumonitis and aspiration pneumonia. N Engl J Med 2001; 344:665–71.
39. Makhnevich A, Feldhamer KH, Kast CL, et al. Aspiration pneumonia in older adults. J Hosp Med 2019;14:429–35.
40. Venkatesan P, Gladman J, Macfarlane JT, et al. A hospital study of community acquired pneumonia in the elderly. Thorax 1990;45(4):254–8.

Advances in the Management of Acute Decompensated Heart Failure

Sumeet S. Mitter, MD, MSc*, Sean P. Pinney, MD

KEYWORDS

- Heart failure with reduced ejection fraction
- Heart failure with preserved ejection fraction • Acute heart failure
- Inpatient management

KEY POINTS

- Heart failure costs are expected to reach $70 billion by 2030. Better assessment of the cause of heart failure is needed to balance quality care and expenditure.
- Without hemodynamic monitoring, congestion and response to decongestive strategies is best assessed with clinical biomarkers and point-of-care lung water assessment.
- Guideline-directed therapy for heart failure with reduced ejection fraction should be initiated or optimized and safe and timely follow-up ensured before discharge to decrease morbidity and mortality.
- Deep phenotyping of heart failure with preserved ejection fraction and diagnosis of suspected cardiac amyloidosis before discharge is paramount given available therapies to reduce heart failure hospitalizations.
- When appropriate, heart team evaluations for transcatheter mitral valve repair or referral for advanced therapies can be considered during hospitalization to improve the prognosis.

EPIDEMIOLOGY

It is estimated that 6.5 million Americans 20 years of age or older are currently living with heart failure and this number is expected to increase to 8 million by 2030.[1] Annual costs for heart failure are expected to increase from $30.7 billion (2010$) to nearly $70 billion by 2030 as well.[1] Moreover, the lifetime risk at age 45 for developing heart failure, through the age of 95 years, is estimated to range between 20% and 45%.[2] At this time, projections from the Get With The Guidelines registry estimate that 50% of cases of hospitalized heart failure will have an ejection fraction of greater than 40%.[3] Left untreated, heart failure with preserved ejection fraction (HFpEF) has

Icahn School of Medicine at Mount Sinai, 1190 5th Avenue, Box 1030, New York, NY 10029, USA
* Corresponding author.
E-mail address: sumeet.mitter@mountsinai.org

Med Clin N Am 104 (2020) 601–614
https://doi.org/10.1016/j.mcna.2020.03.002
0025-7125/20/© 2020 Elsevier Inc. All rights reserved.

medical.theclinics.com

a limited survival of only 35% at 5 years, which is similar to heart failure with reduced ejection fraction (HFrEF).[4] Furthermore, each hospitalization for heart failure yields an increasing risk for 30-day and 1-year mortality.[5] Thus, it is imperative to accurately diagnose, categorize, and manage heart failure given its increasing prevalence, cost, and high fatality rate.

The use of evidence-based, contemporary therapies can change the natural history of heart failure and offers hope for long-term success. This opportunity often begins with an index hospitalization for an acute decompensation from clinical congestion. A challenge for the medical community is to implement such strategies while simultaneously reducing admissions and improving survival. This article reviews the advances in the care of decompensated, hospitalized heart failure (in the absence of cardiogenic shock), including pharmacologic and device management and transitions of care paradigms.

PATHOPHYSIOLOGY

Acute heart failure is a complex disease state. It involves the interplay of neurohormonal activation, hypertension, salt and water retention resulting in vasoconstriction, and increased cardiac filling pressures that result in oxidative stress, inflammation, myocardial injury, impaired renal function, and potential progressive organ damage (**Fig. 1**). Commonly, heart failure is broken into 4 hemodynamic profiles based on organ perfusion (cold or warm) and congestion (dry or wet).[6] Patients admitted with decompensated heart failure usually present with a warm and wet profile, where the

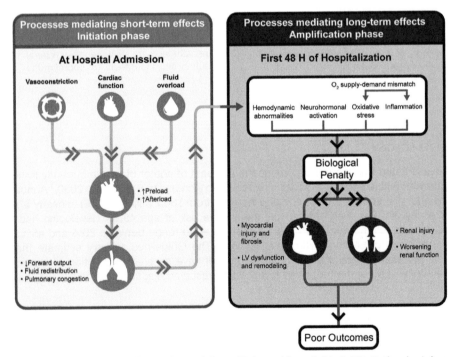

Fig. 1. Pathophysiology of acute heart failure. (*Adapted from* Sabbah HN. Pathophysiology of acute heart failure syndrome: a knowledge gap. Heart Fail Rev 2017;22(6):621-639; with permission.)

pulmonary capillary wedge pressure is elevated with a preserved cardiac index, ensuring intact organ perfusion.[6] The warm and wet profile will be the main focus of this article as opposed to the cold and wet profile, which reflects increased cardiac filling pressures and poor organ perfusion, or cardiogenic shock, that often requires intensive care management.

PATIENT ASSESSMENT

Clinically, patients exhibit congestion or are considered decompensated have evidence of volume overload based on weight; tachypnea; jugular vein distention; pulmonary, abdominal, and peripheral edema with positional and exertional complaints of breathlessness; nausea; early satiety; and fatigue. Although hospitalizations are thought to often be due to a sole event that heralds congestion, acute heart failure in fact is typically not an acute process. Heart failure hospitalizations can be triggered by acute myocardial ischemia, uncontrolled hypertension, arrhythmias, medication and dietary nonadherence, medications that result in negative inotropic activity or sodium retention, acute infections, and/or even worsening valvular heart disease.[7] Data from the Cardio-MEMS (Abbott Laboratories, Lake Bluff, IL) Heart Sensor Allows Monitoring of Pressure to Improve Outcomes in NYHA Class III Heart Failure Patients (CHAMPION) trial in which patients' congestion was managed either with an implantable hemodynamic sensor versus usual reactive responses to patient symptoms and examination noted gradual increases over days in pulmonary arterial pressures on CardioMEMS readings before patients manifested symptoms of worsening congestion.[8]

The 2017 focused update of the 2013 joint guidelines from the American College of Cardiology Foundation and the American Heart Association for the management of heart failure advocate for the assessment of cardiac biomarkers to diagnose, prognosticate and guide therapy for heart failure. This includes a recommendation for the use of brain natriuretic peptide (BNP) (or its precursor N-terminal pro BNP [NTproBNP]) at the time of hospital admission with comparison to outpatient baseline levels for the diagnosis or exclusion of heart failure given their excretion owing to myocardial stretch during congestion.[9,10] Often overlooked is the concomitant recommendation for the comparison of natriuretic peptide levels at the start and end of hospitalization to inform patient prognosis. A decrease in this level by at least 30% is thought to portend a better survival than no change or an increase in levels.[11] This finding is critical, because a decrease in natriuretic peptides as a target of treatment, at least for HFrEF, shows promise based on the inpatient initiation of angiotensin receptor–neprilysin inhibition (ARNI) in the Comparison of Sacubitril-Valsartan versus Enalapril on Effect of NTproBNP in Patients Stabilized from an Acute Heart Failure Episode (PIONEER-HF) trial for optimization of fluid balance and heart failure status.[12] Notably, however, the Effect of Natriuretic Peptide-Guided Therapy on Hospitalization or Cardiovascular Mortality in High Risk Patients with Heart Failure and Reduced Ejection Fraction (GUIDE-IT) trial examining treating toward a specific natriuretic peptide threshold did not find a decrease in heart failure hospitalization and mortality compared with usual care.[13] Other emerging biomarkers predicting heart failure hospitalization and death include ST2 and galectin-3, which may be complimentary to natriuretic peptides as therapeutic targets in the coming years.[10,14,15] ST2 is a member of the IL-1 receptor family and is a marker of myocardial fibrosis and adverse cardiac remodeling. Galectin-3 is secreted by macrophages, mediates cardiac fibrosis, and may identify an advanced heart failure phenotype. Serial decreases in ST2, especially to a target of less than 35 ng/mL, are associated with improved heart failure outcomes, including survival, independent of natriuretic peptides.[16,17]

In addition to serum biomarkers for the assessment for acutely decompensated heart failure, assessment of lung fluid content using the Remote Dielectric Sensing vest (Sensible Medical, Netanya, Israel) has been shown to correlate well with invasive measurements of pulmonary capillary wedge pressure. Decreases in lung fluid content based on the Remote Dielectric Sensing vest may one day serve as a therapeutic target for hospitalized heart failure.[18] Other means of assessing congestion, including the use of handheld point-of-care ultrasound examination to assess lung fluid content, may be more sensitive than biomarker analysis or chest radiographs alone in ruling out decompensated heart failure during the initial examination.[19,20]

Regardless of the strategies used to identify decompensated heart failure, be it physical examination, biomarkers, or point-of-care Remote Dielectric Sensing assessment, the Diuretic Optimization Strategies Evaluation (DOSE) trial showed that worsening renal function may be a trade-off for decongestion but may not necessarily affect postdischarge outcomes, provided there seem to be other objective signs of improvement and the increase is transient.[21] Additionally, small increases in creatinine may accompany up titration of renin–angiotensin system or aldosterone antagonists and hence renal function is not a reliable biomarker to assess decongestion.[22,23] A lack of improvement or worsening of renal function in the setting of what seems to be worsening volume overload despite decongestion may imply patients are in a low cardiac output state, that is, cold and wet, which can be confirmed by use of a Swan-Ganz catheter for assessment of invasive hemodynamics, and would necessitate the use of intravenous vasodilator, inotropic, and/or mechanical support.

TREATMENT
Decongestion

For warm and wet patients, the mainstay of therapy is the use of intravenous loop diuretics. In the setting of severe volume overload, renal venous and splanchnic congestion may decrease the efficacy of a patient's established ambulatory diuretic dose. Hence, per the DOSE trial, a 250% increase in the patient's total ambulatory oral loop diuretic dose given intravenously, in divided doses or as a continuous infusion, should be administered upon inpatient admission to achieve symptom relief.[21] Acute kidney injury from renal venous congestion may improve with diuretic administration because the kidneys are more likely to respond to high -dose diuretics in the setting of a low glomerular filtration rate. In the setting of loop diuretic resistance, oral or intravenous thiazide diuretics can be used to augment diuresis. Target doses and a pathway for escalation of loop and thiazide diuretics are summarized in the 2019 American College of Cardiology Expert Consensus Decision Pathway on Risk Assessment, Management, and Clinical Trajectory of Patients Hospitalized with Heart Failure with a goal of net fluid loss and decrease in weight by ideally at least 1 kg/d (**Table 1**).[7] Limited data suggest that tolvaptan (a vasopressin antagonist) can achieve similar weight loss at 48 hours, despite a lack of improvement in mortality and heart failure hospitalizations in the EVEREST trial.[24,25] The use of vasopressin antagonists may be desirable if there is severe symptomatic hypervolemic hyponatremia with a serum sodium of less than 125 mEq/dL despite fluid restriction to improve heart failure hospitalization morbidity. Other theoretic strategies in the setting of loop diuretic resistance include the adjunctive use of high-dose mineralocorticoid antagonists or even aliquots of hypertonic saline to combat renal sodium retention in the setting of hypochloremia, which may stimulate renin secretion or upregulate sodium chloride channels in the distal convoluted tubule of the kidney.[26]

Table 1
Diuretic dosing

Class	Drug	Usual Inpatient Dosing (Maximum)	Usual Outpatient Dosing (Maximum)
Loop diuretics	Bumetanide	0.5–4.0 mg/h IV once to 3 times daily (5 mg/dose) Or 0.5–2.0 mg/h IV infusion (4 mg/h)	0.5–2.0 mg orally once to twice daily (10 mg/d)
	Furosemide	40–160 mg IV once to 3 times daily (200 mg/dose) Or 5–20 mg/h IV infusion (40 mg/h)	20–80 mg orally once to twice daily (600 mg/d)
	Torsemide	N/A	10–40 mg orally once daily (200 mg/d)
Thiazide-type diuretics	Chlorothiazide	0.5–1 g IV once to twice daily (2 g/d)	N/A
	Hydrochlorothiazide	25–50 mg orally once to twice daily (100 mg/d)	25–50 mg orally once daily (100 mg/d)
	Chlorthalidone	12.5–25 mg orally once to twice daily (100 mg/d)	25–50 mg orally once daily (100 mg/d)
	Metolazone	2.5–5 mg orally once to twice daily (20 mg/d)	2.5–5 mg orally once daily (20 mg/d)

Abbreviation: IV, intravenously.

From Hollenberg SM, Warner Stevenson L, Ahmad T, et al. 2019 ACC expert consensus decision pathway on risk assessment, management, and clinical trajectory of patients hospitalized with heart failure: A report of the American College of Cardiology solution set oversight committee. J Am Coll Cardiol 2019;74(15):1981; with permission.

Adjunctive Therapies

Inotropic or parenteral vasodilator assisted diuresis is not supported by clear evidence for warm and wet patients. The Renal Optimization Strategies Evaluation (ROSE) acute heart failure trial tested the addition of low-dose dopamine or low-dose nesiritide to improve symptoms of congestion while preserving renal function, however, did not find a benefit.[27] If attempts to decongest a patient are unsuccessful with intensification of intravenous diuretic strategies, in appropriately selected patients and in conjunction with nephrology, ultrafiltration can be pursued for decongestion by mobilizing plasma water and solute across a semipermeable membrane while maintaining intravascular volume.[9] Careful consideration with regard to resource management and the need for central venous access, nursing services, and anticoagulation are needed when pursuing ultrafiltration.

Hospitalizations for acutely decompensated heart failure are an opportunity to address comorbid noncardiac diseases that may improve the quality of life for patients with heart failure. The 2017 focused update of the heart failure guidelines incorporated the best available data to make recommendations on the management of anemia and sleep-disordered breathing among patients with heart failure. Intravenous iron replacement for iron deficient chronic anemia (ferritin <100 ng/mL or 100–300 ng/mL if transferrin saturation is <20% for patients with New York Heart Association [NYHA] functional class II and III heart failure) can be considered based on limited data from 2 trials examining the use of ferric carboxymaltose to improve NYHA functional class and 6-minute walk distance tests.[10,28,29] Clinical trials are being conducted with novel intravenous iron formulations to confirm improvements in morbidity and assess the impact on mortality. Furthermore, formal sleep testing as an inpatient or outpatient should be pursued for patients with NYHA functional class II to IV heart failure for whom there is suspicion for sleep-disordered breathing. A sleep study can differentiate between central and obstructive sleep apnea and facilitate initiation of continuous positive airway pressure to improve sleep quality and nocturnal oxygenation.[10]

Guideline-Directed Therapy for Heart Failure with Reduced Ejection Fraction

Among patients with an ejection fraction of less than 40% hospitalized for heart failure it is imperative to continue guideline-directed medial therapy (GDMT) for heart failure to maintain neurohormonal antagonism. Furthermore, as patients approach clinical euvolemia during the decongestion phase of a hospitalization for heart failure, it is crucial to uptitrate or initiate GDMT because it provides an opportunity to optimize dosing regimens that often can take a considerable amount of time as an outpatient and improve outcomes after discharge.[30] Target doses of neurohormonal antagonists and a pathway for escalation are summarized in the 2017 American College of Cardiology Expert Consensus Decision Pathway for Optimization of Heart Failure Treatment.[31] Recent data from the Change in Management of Patients with Heart Failure (CHAMP-HF) registry suggest that less than 1% of patients are on target doses of GDMT over a period of 12 months in the outpatient setting.[32] This finding implies significant undermanagement of patients with chronic HFrEF, which may begin in the prehospital discharge setting.

For many years the mainstay of chronic HFrEF management used a 3-pronged, evidence-based approach of neurohormonal antagonism to improve mortality (**Table 2**):

- Angiotensin-converting enzyme inhibitors (ACEi) or angiotensin receptor blockers (ARB) for those who cannot tolerate ACEi per the SOLVD and CHARM-Alternative studies, respectively[33,34];

Table 2
Cumulative impact of evidence-based HFrEF therapies

	Relative Risk Reduction (%)	Iterative 2-Year Mortality (%)
None	—	35
ACEi or ARB	23	27
Beta-blocker	35	18
Aldosterone antagonists	30	13
ARNI (replacing ACEi or ARB)	16	10.9
SGLT2i	17	9.1
CRT-D (EF ≤35%; QRS duration ≥120 ms)	36	5.8

Cumulative risk reduction if all evidence-based medical therapies are used: relative risk reduction, 83.4%; absolute risk reduction, 29.2%; number needed to treat, 3.4.

Abbreviations: CRT-D, cardiac resynchronization therapy; EF, ejection fraction; SGLT2i, sodium-glucose cotransporter-2 inhibitors.

Data from Fonarow GC, Yancy CW, Hernandez AF, et al. Potential impact of optimal implementation of evidence-based heart failure therapies on mortality. Am Heart J 2011;161(6):1024-1030; and Fonarow GC. Statins and n-3 fatty acid supplementation in heart failure. Lancet 2008;372(9645):1195-1196.

- Beta blockers, namely, carvedilol, metoprolol succinate, and bisoprolol, per the US Carvedilol Study, MERIT-HF and CIBIS-II studies, respectively[35–37]; and
- Aldosterone antagonism with either spironolactone or eplerenone per the RALES and EMPHASIS-HF studies, respectively.[38,39]

The 2019 American College of Cardiology expert consensus pathway for patients hospitalized for heart failure underscores the initiation or dose optimization of these agents before hospital discharge.[7] The PARADIGM-HF trial established the superiority of sacubitril/valsartan to enalapril among patients with ambulatory heart failure with an ejection fraction of less than 35% in decreasing cardiovascular death and heart failure hospitalizations.[40] If minimum doses of ACEi or ARB are hemodynamically tolerated, transition to an ARNI is preferred to achieve such mortality benefit (see **Table 2**). The recommendation to initiate or transition to an ARNI is reflected in the heart failure guidelines and consensus statements for heart failure management.[7,10,31] Hospitalization for acutely decompensated heart failure provides an opportunity to shift the needle on transitioning from ACEi or ARB to an ARNI before hospital discharge. Among hospitalized patients, the PIONEER-HF study was notable for sustained greater decreases in NTproBNP among patients initiated on ARNI versus ACEi during and after hospitalizations.[12] The push to initiate this transition to an ARNI as early as possible is furthermore reinforced by the PROVE-HF study demonstrating improvements in reverse cardiac remodeling and myocardial structure as NTproBNP levels are lowered with exposure to an ARNI.[41]

Optimization of GDMT during an index or subsequent hospitalization for heart failure also provides an opportunity to address medication adjustments in select populations. Per the A-HEFT study, the addition of hydralazine and isosorbide dinitrate to optimal doses of ACEi and beta-blockers in self-identified African Americans is recommended.[9,42] This finding reflects a 43% relative risk reduction in mortality and number needed to treat of 21 to prevent 1 death compared with placebo.[42,43] The 2013 heart failure guidelines also recommend considering the combination of hydralazine and isosorbide dinitrate in lieu of an ACEi or ARB in any individual who cannot tolerate such agents owing to drug intolerance, renal insufficiency, hypotension, or hyperkalemia.[9] Among patients with HFrEF with NYHA functional class II symptoms or more, in sinus rhythm and a heart rate of greater than 70 despite maximally tolerated doses of evidence-based beta-blockers, the predischarge time period during a heart failure hospitalization provides an opportunity to introduce ivabradine given its ability to reduce heart failure hospitalizations and morbidity.[10,44] The next iteration of the heart failure guidelines will likely reflect the role of sodium-glucose cotransporter-2 inhibitors in decreasing mortality and heart failure hospitalizations for all comers with heart failure, irrespective of hemoglobin A1c, given the recent DAPA-HF trial results.[45] This strategy will move optimal GDMT for HFrEF from including at least 3 drug classes (ACEi/ARB or ARNI, beta-blockers and aldosterone antagonists) to at least 4 drug classes that could also begin in the hospital.[46]

Although not essential to inpatient management, discussions regarding the use of implantable cardioverter defibrillators, cardiac synchronization therapy, and percutaneous repair of mitral regurgitation can be initiated before discharge. Consultation of the electrophysiology service can be considered for implantable cardiac defibrillator therapy for patients with HFrEF with an ejection fraction of less than 35% to prevent sudden cardiac death, or for implantation of cardiac resynchronization therapy for individuals with an ejection fraction of less than 35%, left bundle branch and QRS duration of greater than 150 milliseconds, and residual heart failure symptoms despite being on maximally tolerated heart failure medications for at least 3 months.[9] Patients with HFrEF and residual severe functional mitral regurgitation with persistent heart failure symptoms or hospitalizations despite being on maximally tolerated GDMT and adequate decongestion and potential use of cardiac resynchronization therapy should be referred for evaluation by a heart team, including an advanced heart failure cardiologist, structural cardiologist, and cardiothoracic surgeon for consideration of percutaneous edge-to-edge mitral valve repair. The COAPT trial found a 38% relative decrease in all-cause mortality and a 47% decrease in hospitalizations after 2 years with the use of transcatheter mitral valve repair after optimization of GDMT.[47] Other considerations by a heart team in this setting may include advanced therapies, such as a left ventricular assist device or heart transplant, particularly for patients deemed to have a poor prognosis despite efforts to optimize medical and device therapy.

Phenotypic Management of Heart Failure with Preserved Ejection Fraction

The 2013 heart failure guidelines define HFpEF as an ejection fraction of greater than 50%.[9] The increasing burden of HFpEF, especially among the elderly, necessitates proper phenotyping of disease to deliver appropriate therapy in this setting. To date, clinical trials for HFpEF have failed to yield medical therapy that has a shown a mortality benefit. Nonetheless, given that 50% of hospitalized heart failure is now attributed to HFpEF, it is imperative to implement therapy to reduce heart failure hospitalization and morbidity given the significant financial burden and impairment to quality of life. In the absence of an infiltrative cardiomyopathy leading to a HFpEF syndrome, the American College of Cardiology Foundation/American Heart Association Task Force heart failure guidelines emphasize the management of comorbid cardiovascular conditions that contribute to a HFpEF syndrome, all of which can be addressed during a hospitalization for acute decompensation. These factors include recommendations for decongestion with diuretics and adequate blood pressure control according to clinical practice guidelines, as well as recommendations for potential coronary revascularization in the setting of myocardial ischemia and rate and rhythm control of atrial fibrillation.[9] Moreover, results from the TOPCAT trial have resulted in the recommendation of aldosterone antagonists to decrease heart hospitalizations in individuals with heart failure, an ejection fraction of greater than 45% and an estimated glomerular filtration rate of greater than 30 mL/min, a serum creatinine of less than 2.5 mg/dL, and potassium of less than 5.0 mEq/L.[10,48] Not all HFpEF syndromes can be managed with a single therapy, which reflects the heterogenous nature of a syndrome that often includes comorbid myocardial disease, chronic kidney disease, obesity, impaired lung mechanics, and reduced skeletal muscle reserve.[49,50] After decongestion, an examination of clinical characteristics and the use of advanced echocardiography to assess myocardial mechanics and strain/deformation imaging can shed light on various phenogroups of the umbrella diagnosis of HFpEF. Identifying impaired myocardial relaxation, cardiometabolic impairments, and cardiorenal syndrome with poor right ventricular mechanics can guide potential therapies.[51] Shah and colleagues[52] have proposed an iterative framework for the management of various HFpEF syndromes that reflects clinical characteristics and comorbid noncardiac and cardiac diagnoses that can help to optimize therapy (**Table 3**).

Recent results of the PARAGON-HF trial comparing sacubitril/valsartan to valsartan in HFpEF patients with an ejection fraction of 45% or greater did not show a statistical decrease in mortality and heart failure hospitalizations.[53] Nonetheless, the trial did elucidate potential differences in response to therapy based on gender and ejection fraction ranges. Women and those with an ejection fraction of 45% to 57% (less than the median in the study), seemed to derive a greater benefit.[53] Older men with HFpEF are increasingly being recognized to have transthyretin cardiac amyloidosis, which may explain the lack of benefit from an ARNI in the trial.[54] Furthermore, patients with a lower ejection fraction in the trial may reflect patients transitioning to HFrEF and have more neurohormonal activation, for whom ARNIs may provide more physiologic and structural benefit.[55]

The possibility of inclusion of many patients with transthyretin amyloidosis in HFpEF trials, as recently as PARAGON-HF, further emphasizes the need for deep phenotyping of HFpEF during admissions for acutely decompensated heart failure, whereby the use of precision medicine, advanced imaging, and genotypic information can further clarify phenotypic manifestations of disease. For example, one contemporary series predicts that nearly 15% of hospitalized HFpEF patients with left ventricular hypertrophy have wild-type transthyretin cardiac amyloidosis.[56] Advanced cardiac imaging using strain echocardiography, cardiac MRI, and technetium pyrophosphate scanning during admission for acutely decompensated heart failure can help to diagnose transthyretin cardiac amyloidosis in these cases. This strategy is critical, given the results of the ATTR-ACT study, which demonstrated an improvement in all-cause mortality and cardiovascular hospitalization for tafamidis compared with placebo for patients with transthyretin cardiac amyloidosis.[57]

SAFE TRANSITIONS IN CARE

After decongestion, deep phenotyping and optimization of heart failure therapies for both HFrEF and HFpEF, patients are vulnerable and at high risk for rehospitalization soon after discharge, with some estimates as high as 25% within 30 days. The implementation of robust transitions in care programs may be effective in decreasing heart failure rehospitalizations. Before discharge, best care practices include assessment of cardiac biomarkers and potentially lung water content, ensuring that discharge medications reflect GDMT, medication teaching, and nutrition counseling. After discharge, expert consensus recommends follow-up by phone within 48 to 72 hours of discharge to assess for any gaps in care and to ensure follow-up by a heart failure

Table 3
Phenotypic-specific HFpEF treatment strategy using a matrix of predisposition phenotypes and clinical presentation phenotypes

HFpEF predisposition phenotypes	HFpEF Clinical Presentation Phenotypes				
	Lung Congestion	+ Chronotropic Incompetence	+ Pulmonary Hypertension (CpcPH)	+ Skeletal Muscle Weakness	+ Atrial Fibrillation
Overweight/obesity/metabolic syndrome/type 2 DM	**Diuretics (loop diuretic in DM)** **Caloric restriction** Statins Inorganic nitrite/nitrate Sacubitril Spironolactone	+Rate adaptive atrial pacing	+Pulmonary vasodilators (eg, PDE5I)	+ **Exercise training program**	+Cardioversion +Rate control + **Anticoagulation**
+ Arterial hypertension	+ACEI/ARB	+ACEI/ARB +Rate adaptive atrial pacing	+ACEI/ARB +Pulmonary vasodilators (eg, PDE5I)	+ACEI/ARB + **Exercise training program**	+ACEI/ARB +Cardioversion +Rate control + **Anticoagulation**
+ Renal dysfunction	+Ultrafiltration if needed	+Ultrafiltration if needed +Rate adaptive atrial pacing	+Ultrafiltration if needed +Pulmonary vasodilators (eg, PDE5I)	+Ultrafiltration if needed + **Exercise training program**	+Ultrafiltration if needed +Cardioversion +Rate control + **Anticoagulation**
+ CAD	+ACEI + Revascularization	+ACEI + Revascularization +Rate adaptive atrial pacing	+ACEI + Revascularization +Pulmonary vasodilators (eg, PDE5I)	+ACEI + Revascularization + **Exercise training program**	+ACEI + Revascularization +Cardioversion +Rate control + **Anticoagulation**

Abbreviations: CAD, coronary artery disease; CpcPH, combined precapillary and postcapillary pulmonary hypertension; DM, diabetes mellitus; PDE5I, phosphodiesterase-5 inhibitor.

Adapted from Shah SJ, Kitzman DW, Borlaug BA, et al. Phenotype-Specific Treatment of Heart Failure With Preserved Ejection Fraction: A Multiorgan Roadmap. Circulation 2016;134(1):73-90; with permission.

specialist within 7 to 14 days of discharge.[7] During hospital follow-up, the focus should be on delivering quality care to improve survival rather than merely preventing a readmission. The Centers for Medicare & Medicaid Services' Hospital Readmissions Reduction Program for heart failure may be associated with an increase the 30-day risk-adjusted mortality that continues to increase over time.[58,59] A restructuring of quality metrics is needed given the potential harm associated with emphasizing readmissions reduction. Further work is needed to balance decongestion, optimization of GDMT, and safe transitions to decrease readmissions and, ultimately, mortality.

SUMMARY

The burden of acutely decompensated heart failure requiring admission has changed, now reflecting an increasing prevalence of HFpEF syndromes. Although the natural history of HFrEF has changed with the initiation of at least triple agent GDMT, an increased focus on understanding the determinants of congestion and how to adequately decongest a patient may lead to fewer hospitalizations for heart failure. The use of biomarkers and point-of-care lung water assessment helps to assess for improved hemodynamic congestion at the end of a hospitalization. Ensuring optimal medical and device therapy for HFrEF and close follow-up in the vulnerable phase after hospital discharge may ensure therapeutic success. A shift toward the use of quadruple therapy for HFrEF with sodium-glucose cotransporter-2 inhibitors and use of transcatheter therapies for mitral valve repair in carefully selected patients offers the potential for additional benefit. Furthermore, deep phenotyping of HFpEF, including cardiac amyloidosis, results in appropriate therapy assignments for a heterogenous syndrome. The focus should remain on the patient to ensure therapeutic success, and mortality improvement while avoiding the potential unintended consequences from quality measurement programs.

DISCLOSURE

S.S. Mitter reports being on the Speaker's Bureau for Abbott Laboratories, and receiving Honoraria from Cowen & Co. S.P. Pinney reports consulting for Abbott Laboratories, CareDx, Medtronic, Inc, and Procyrion.

REFERENCES

1. Virani SS, Alonso A, Benjamin EJ, et al. Heart disease and stroke statistics-2020 update: a report from the American Heart Association. Circulation 2020;141(9):e139–596.

2. Huffman MD, Berry JD, Ning H, et al. Lifetime risk for heart failure among white and Black Americans: cardiovascular lifetime risk pooling project. J Am Coll Cardiol 2013;61(14):1510–7.

3. Oktay AA, Rich JD, Shah SJ. The emerging epidemic of heart failure with preserved ejection fraction. Curr Heart Fail Rep 2013;10(4):401–10.

4. Owan TE, Hodge DO, Herges RM, et al. Trends in prevalence and outcome of heart failure with preserved ejection fraction. N Engl J Med 2006;355(3):251–9.

5. Setoguchi S, Stevenson LW, Schneeweiss S. Repeated hospitalizations predict mortality in the community population with heart failure. Am Heart J 2007; 154(2):260–6.

6. Nohria A, Lewis E, Stevenson LW. Medical management of advanced heart failure. JAMA 2002;287(5):628–40.

7. Hollenberg SM, Warner Stevenson L, Ahmad T, et al. 2019 ACC expert consensus decision pathway on risk assessment, management, and clinical trajectory of patients hospitalized with heart failure: a report of the American College of Cardiology Solution Set Oversight Committee. J Am Coll Cardiol 2019;74(15): 1966–2011.

8. Abraham WT, Adamson PB, Bourge RC, et al. Wireless pulmonary artery haemodynamic monitoring in chronic heart failure: a randomised controlled trial. Lancet 2011;377(9766):658–66.

9. Yancy CW, Jessup M, Bozkurt B, et al. 2013 ACCF/AHA guideline for the management of heart failure: a report of the American College of Cardiology Foundation/American Heart Association Task Force on Practice Guidelines. J Am Coll Cardiol 2013;62(16):e147–239.

10. Yancy CW, Jessup M, Bozkurt B, et al. 2017 ACC/AHA/HFSA focused update of the 2013 ACCF/AHA guideline for the management of heart failure: a report of the American College of Cardiology/American Heart Association Task Force on Clinical Practice Guidelines and the Heart Failure Society of America. J Am Coll Cardiol 2017;70(6):776–803.

11. Stienen S, Salah K, Moons AH, et al. NT-proBNP (N-Terminal pro-B-Type Natriuretic Peptide)-guided therapy in acute decompensated heart failure: PRIMA II Randomized Controlled Trial (Can NT-ProBNP-guided therapy during hospital admission for acute decompensated heart failure reduce mortality and readmissions?). Circulation 2018;137(16):1671–83.

12. Velazquez EJ, Morrow DA, DeVore AD, et al. Angiotensin-neprilysin inhibition in acute decompensated heart failure. N Engl J Med 2019;380(6):539–48.

13. Felker GM, Anstrom KJ, Adams KF, et al. Effect of natriuretic peptide-guided therapy on hospitalization or cardiovascular mortality in high-risk patients with heart failure and reduced ejection fraction: a randomized clinical trial. JAMA 2017; 318(8):713–20.

14. Felker GM, Fiuzat M, Thompson V, et al. Soluble ST2 in ambulatory patients with heart failure: association with functional capacity and long-term outcomes. Circ Heart Fail 2013;6(6):1172–9.

15. Felker GM, Fiuzat M, Shaw LK, et al. Galectin-3 in ambulatory patients with heart failure: results from the HF-ACTION study. Circ Heart Fail 2012;5(1):72–8.

16. Breidthardt T, Balmelli C, Twerenbold R, et al. Heart failure therapy-induced early ST2 changes may offer long-term therapy guidance. J Card Fail 2013;19(12): 821–8.

17. Gaggin HK, Szymonifka J, Bhardwaj A, et al. Head-to-head comparison of serial soluble ST2, growth differentiation factor-15, and highly-sensitive troponin T measurements in patients with chronic heart failure. JACC Heart Fail 2014;2(1):65–72.

18. Uriel N, Sayer G, Imamura T, et al. Relationship between noninvasive assessment of lung fluid volume and invasively measured cardiac hemodynamics. J Am Heart Assoc 2018;7(22):e009175.

19. Pivetta E, Goffi A, Nazerian P, et al. Lung ultrasound integrated with clinical assessment for the diagnosis of acute decompensated heart failure in the emergency department: a randomized controlled trial. Eur J Heart Fail 2019;21(6): 754–66.

20. Buessler A, Chouihed T, Duarte K, et al. Accuracy of several lung ultrasound methods for the diagnosis of acute heart failure in the ED: a multicenter prospective study. Chest 2020;157(1):99–110.

21. Felker GM, Lee KL, Bull DA, et al. Diuretic strategies in patients with acute decompensated heart failure. N Engl J Med 2011;364(9):797–805.

22. Testani JM, Cappola TP, McCauley BD, et al. Impact of worsening renal function during the treatment of decompensated heart failure on changes in renal function during subsequent hospitalization. Am Heart J 2011;161(5):944–9.

23. Vardeny O, Wu DH, Desai A, et al. Influence of baseline and worsening renal function on efficacy of spironolactone in patients with severe heart failure: insights from RALES (Randomized Aldactone Evaluation Study). J Am Coll Cardiol 2012; 60(20):2082–9.

24. Cox ZL, Hung R, Lenihan DJ, et al. Diuretic strategies for loop diuretic resistance in acute heart failure: the 3T trial. JACC Heart Fail 2019;8(3):157–68.

25. Konstam MA, Gheorghiade M, Burnett JC Jr, et al. Effects of oral tolvaptan in patients hospitalized for worsening heart failure: the EVEREST Outcome Trial. JAMA 2007;297(12):1319–31.

26. Griffin M, Soufer A, Goljo E, et al. Real world use of hypertonic saline in refractory acute decompensated heart failure: a U.S. center's experience. JACC Heart Fail 2020;8(3):199–208.

27. Chen HH, Anstrom KJ, Givertz MM, et al. Low-dose dopamine or low-dose nesiritide in acute heart failure with renal dysfunction: the ROSE acute heart failure randomized trial. JAMA 2013;310(23):2533–43.

28. Anker SD, Comin Colet J, Filippatos G, et al. Ferric carboxymaltose in patients with heart failure and iron deficiency. N Engl J Med 2009;361(25):2436–48.

29. Ponikowski P, van Veldhuisen DJ, Comin-Colet J, et al. Beneficial effects of long-term intravenous iron therapy with ferric carboxymaltose in patients with symptomatic heart failure and iron deficiency dagger. Eur Heart J 2015;36(11):657–68.

30. Tran RH, Aldemerdash A, Chang P, et al. Guideline-directed medical therapy and survival following hospitalization in patients with heart failure. Pharmacotherapy 2018;38(4):406–16.

31. Yancy CW, Januzzi JL Jr, Allen LA, et al. 2017 ACC expert consensus decision pathway for optimization of heart failure treatment: answers to 10 pivotal issues about heart failure with reduced ejection fraction: a report of the American College of Cardiology Task Force on Expert Consensus Decision Pathways. J Am Coll Cardiol 2018;71(2):201–30.

32. Greene SJ, Fonarow GC, DeVore AD, et al. Titration of medical therapy for heart failure with reduced ejection fraction. J Am Coll Cardiol 2019;73(19):2365–83.

33. Investigators S, Yusuf S, Pitt B, et al. Effect of enalapril on survival in patients with reduced left ventricular ejection fractions and congestive heart failure. N Engl J Med 1991;325(5):293–302.

34. Cohn JN, Tognoni G. Valsartan Heart Failure Trial I. A randomized trial of the angiotensin-receptor blocker valsartan in chronic heart failure. N Engl J Med 2001;345(23):1667–75.

35. Packer M, Bristow MR, Cohn JN, et al. The effect of carvedilol on morbidity and mortality in patients with chronic heart failure. U.S. Carvedilol Heart Failure Study Group. N Engl J Med 1996;334(21):1349–55.

36. Effect of metoprolol CR/XL in chronic heart failure: Metoprolol CR/XL Randomised Intervention Trial in Congestive Heart Failure (MERIT-HF). Lancet 1999;353(9169): 2001–7.

37. The Cardiac Insufficiency Bisoprolol Study II (CIBIS-II): a randomised trial. Lancet 1999;353(9146):9–13.

38. Pitt B, Zannad F, Remme WJ, et al. The effect of spironolactone on morbidity and mortality in patients with severe heart failure. Randomized Aldactone Evaluation Study Investigators. N Engl J Med 1999;341(10):709–17.

39. Zannad F, McMurray JJ, Krum H, et al. Eplerenone in patients with systolic heart failure and mild symptoms. N Engl J Med 2011;364(1):11–21.

40. McMurray JJ, Packer M, Desai AS, et al. Angiotensin-neprilysin inhibition versus enalapril in heart failure. N Engl J Med 2014;371(11):993–1004.

41. Januzzi JL Jr, Prescott MF, Butler J, et al. Association of Change in N-Terminal Pro-B-type natriuretic peptide following initiation of sacubitril-valsartan treatment with cardiac structure and function in patients with heart failure with reduced ejection fraction. JAMA 2019;322(11):1085–95.

42. Taylor AL, Ziesche S, Yancy C, et al. Combination of isosorbide dinitrate and hydralazine in blacks with heart failure. N Engl J Med 2004;351(20):2049–57.

43. Fonarow GC, Hernandez AF, Solomon SD, et al. Potential mortality reduction with optimal implementation of angiotensin receptor neprilysin inhibitor therapy in heart failure. JAMA Cardiol 2016;1(6):714–7.

44. Swedberg K, Komajda M, Bohm M, et al. Ivabradine and outcomes in chronic heart failure (SHIFT): a randomised placebo-controlled study. Lancet 2010; 376(9744):875–85.

45. McMurray JJV, Solomon SD, Inzucchi SE, et al. Dapagliflozin in patients with heart failure and reduced ejection fraction. N Engl J Med 2019;381(21):1995–2008.

46. Felker GM. Building the foundation for a new era of quadruple therapy in heart failure. Circulation 2020;141(2):112–4.

47. Stone GW, Lindenfeld J, Abraham WT, et al. Transcatheter mitral-valve repair in patients with heart failure. N Engl J Med 2018;379(24):2307–18.

48. Pitt B, Pfeffer MA, Assmann SF, et al. Spironolactone for heart failure with preserved ejection fraction. N Engl J Med 2014;370(15):1383–92.

49. Kitzman DW, Shah SJ. The HFpEF obesity phenotype: the elephant in the room. J Am Coll Cardiol 2016;68(2):200–3.

50. Borlaug BA. The pathophysiology of heart failure with preserved ejection fraction. Nat Rev Cardiol 2014;11(9):507–15.

51. Shah SJ, Katz DH, Selvaraj S, et al. Phenomapping for novel classification of heart failure with preserved ejection fraction. Circulation 2015;131(3):269–79.

52. Shah SJ, Kitzman DW, Borlaug BA, et al. Phenotype-specific treatment of heart failure with preserved ejection fraction: a multiorgan roadmap. Circulation 2016;134(1):73–90.

53. Solomon SD, McMurray JJV, Anand IS, et al. Angiotensin-neprilysin inhibition in heart failure with preserved ejection fraction. N Engl J Med 2019;381(17): 1609–20.

54. McMurray JJV, Jackson AM, Lam CSP, et al. Effects of sacubitril-valsartan, versus valsartan, in women compared to men with heart failure and preserved ejection fraction: insights from PARAGON-HF. Circulation 2020;141(5):338–51.

55. Solomon SD, Vaduganathan M, Claggett BL, et al. Sacubitril/valsartan across the spectrum of ejection fraction in heart failure. Circulation 2020;141(5):352–61.

56. Gonzalez-Lopez E, Gallego-Delgado M, Guzzo-Merello G, et al. Wild-type transthyretin amyloidosis as a cause of heart failure with preserved ejection fraction. Eur Heart J 2015;36(38):2585–94.

57. Maurer MS, Schwartz JH, Gundapaneni B, et al. Tafamidis treatment for patients with transthyretin amyloid cardiomyopathy. N Engl J Med 2018;379(11):1007–16.

58. Dharmarajan K, Wang Y, Lin Z, et al. Association of changing hospital readmission rates with mortality rates after hospital discharge. JAMA 2017;318(3):270–8.

59. Vaduganathan M, McCarthy CP, Ayers C, et al. Longitudinal trajectories of hospital performance across targeted cardiovascular conditions in the USA. Eur Heart J Qual Care Clin Outcomes 2020;6(1):62–71.

Recent Advances in the Management of Acute Exacerbations of Chronic Obstructive Pulmonary Disease

Stacey-Ann Whittaker Brown, MD, MPH*,
Sidney Braman, MD, Master FCCP

KEYWORDS

- COPD exacerbation • Assessment • Risk factors • Prevention

KEY POINTS

- AECOPD usually results from viral or bacterial respiratory infections, but may also result from exposure to environmental pollution.
- Treatment of patients admitted with AECOPD involves antibiotics in select patients with increased sputum volume or purulence, corticosteroids, and short-acting bronchodilator therapy.
- Noninvasive positive pressure ventilation is recommended as first-line treatment of patients presenting with acute or acute-on-chronic hypercapnic respiratory failure if no contraindications exist. It is also beneficial in the postexacerbation period in patients with persistent hypercapnia.
- The following interventions are associated with reduced exacerbations or mortality: long-term oxygen therapy or NIPPV based on physiologic parameters, smoking cessation counseling, pharmacologic therapies including long-acting bronchodilators and inhaled corticosteroids, antibiotic therapy or selective phosphodiesterase-4 inhibitor use in those with frequent or history of severe exacerbations, and vaccination.

DEFINITION AND EPIDEMIOLOGY

Chronic obstructive pulmonary disease (COPD) is a chronic, irreversible obstructive lung disease that results from exposure to noxious stimuli, such as tobacco smoke and air pollution.[1] Fourteen million Americans have COPD,[2] with an estimated global prevalence of 328 million.[3] It is the third leading cause of death worldwide.[4] Symptomatically, it is manifested by chronic dyspnea and/or sputum production and subtypes

Division of Pulmonary, Critical Care and Sleep Medicine, Icahn School of Medicine at Mount Sinai, One Gustave L. Levy Place, Box 1232, New York, NY 10029, USA
* Corresponding author.
E-mail address: stacey-ann.brown@mountsinai.org

Med Clin N Am 104 (2020) 615–630
https://doi.org/10.1016/j.mcna.2020.02.003

include predominantly emphysema, chronic bronchitis, or both. It requires spirometric confirmation of fixed airflow obstruction, defined as a forced expiratory volume in 1 second (FEV_1)/forced vital capacity ratio of less than 70% predicted, after the administration of a short-acting bronchodilator.

The acute exacerbation of COPD (AECOPD) is defined as "an acute worsening of respiratory symptoms that result in additional therapy."[1] A severe exacerbation is any requiring emergency room consultation or hospitalization. Severe exacerbations account for 1.5 million emergency room visits and 699,000 hospitalizations in the United States annually.[2]

The severity of COPD is an interplay of pulmonary function, symptom burden, and exacerbation history. The strongest independent risk factor for an acute exacerbation is a history of exacerbation.[5] Current guidelines as outlined by the Global Initiative of Chronic Obstructive Lung Disease (GOLD) strategy favor assessing COPD along two independent measures: lung function (as defined by FEV_1% predicted and graded on a numeric scale 1–4), and a combination of symptoms and exacerbations (along an alphabetical scale ABCD) (**Fig. 1**).[1] For the latter, symptom burden is assessed using the modified British Medical Research Council Questionnaire scale[6] and/or the COPD Assessment Tool.[7] High-risk exacerbation history is defined as one or more resulting in a hospital admission and/or two or more exacerbations in the past year. Patients admitted with an AECOPD are by definition group C or group D.

GOLD Stage	Post-bronchodilator FEV1, % predicted
I- Mild	= 80
II- Moderate	50–79
III-Severe	30–49
IV-Very Severe	<30

High Risk Exacerbation History
- At least 1 hospitalization OR
- ≥2 moderate to severe exacerbations

Low Risk Exacerbation History
- No hospitalizations AND
- <2 moderate to severe exacerbations

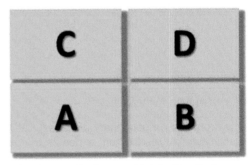

Low Symptom Burden
- mMRC<2
- CAT<10

High Symptom Burden
- mMRC≥2
- CAT≥10

Fig. 1. The GOLD assessment for COPD. A patient with COPD with a post-bronchodilator FEV_1 of 40% who was very symptomatic (CAT score = 15) and only one exacerbation in the past year (without hospitalization) is GOLD stage 3, group B. Management is determined by ABCD group, not spirometric stage. CAT, COPD assessment test; mMRC, modified British Medical Research Council Questionnaire. (*Adapted from* Global Strategy for the Diagnosis, Management, and Prevention of Chronic Obstructive Pulmonary Disease 2020 Report. Global Initiative for Chronic Obstructive Lung Disease (GOLD). Available at: https://goldcopd.org/wp-content/uploads/2019/11/GOLD-2020-REPORT-ver1.0wms.pdf. Accessed Feb 7 2020; with permission.)

CAUSES

Acute exacerbations are caused by complex interactions that involve preexisting airway inflammation and an enhanced inflammatory burden caused by host defenses to infection and environmental insults.

Viral Infections

Viral infections account for 43% of exacerbations.[8] Exacerbations triggered by respiratory viral infections are more severe, have longer recovery times, are associated with higher levels of inflammatory markers, and are more likely to result in hospital readmission.[9,10] The most frequently detected viral species are[11]

- Human rhinovirus (16%)
- Respiratory syncytial virus (10%)
- Influenza (7%)
- Coronavirus (4%)
- Adenovirus (2%)
- Human metapneumovirus (2%)

Since the introduction of influenza immunization, this virus has become a less prominent cause of exacerbation, although it is still likely to be an important factor at times of epidemics.

Bacterial Infections

The precise role of bacteria during COPD exacerbations has been difficult to assess as a result of airway bacterial colonization. Wang and colleagues[12] have discussed an important paradox in COPD: despite the accumulation of leukocytes in the airways with increasing disease severity, there is still a major failure to adequately control and eradicate respiratory pathogens. Nearly 50% of patients with COPD are colonized with pathogenic bacteria, such as *Haemophilus influenzae*, *Streptococcus pneumoniae*, and *Moraxella catarrhalis*.[10,12-14] AECOPD complicated by bacterial infection enhances neutrophilic inflammation and this results in increased levels of neutrophil elastase, tumor necrosis factor-α, and interleukin-8; the elastase produced by neutrophils inhibits tracheobronchial ciliary function, and contributes to impaired bacterial clearance.[15,16] In addition, secondary bacterial infection following viral infection is common and accounts for one-quarter of infective exacerbations.[17]

Environmental Pollution

AECOPD has been associated with increased concentrations of ambient air pollutants, such as fine particulate matter with a diameter of less than 2.5 μm nitric oxide, and sulfur dioxide,[18] and is seen mainly in large industrial cities. Numerous personal devices have recently been developed to help patients with COPD or other respiratory diseases monitor ambient air pollution and prevent air-pollution-related COPD exacerbations.[19]

CLINICAL PRESENTATION AND ASSESSMENT
Presenting Symptoms

Some authors have defined AECOPD as the presence for at least 2 consecutive days of increase in any two major symptoms or increase in one major and one minor symptom,[20,21] although international consensus defines AECOPD as any combination of these symptoms warranting treatment.[1]

Major symptoms include
- Dyspnea
- Sputum purulence
- Increased sputum volume

Minor symptoms include
- Wheeze
- Sore throat
- Cough
- Nasal congestion

Acute respiratory acidosis occurs in 20% of patients, and 50% present with hypoxemia (saturation <90%).[22]

Assessment

COPD frequently coexists with other medical conditions.[23] Decompensated heart failure, ischemic heart disease, and thromboembolism may mimic an AECOPD. Outlined in **Box 1** are the recommended tests in the initial evaluation of an AECOPD presenting to the emergency room.

Chest radiography is recommended because there are substantial rates of abnormalities in chest radiography among patients with an AECOPD; one study reported chest radiograph findings prompted change in management in 24% of patients.[24] In addition to unsuspected pulmonary infiltrates, new lung masses, pneumothorax, and evidence of pulmonary edema can be seen.[25]

Another useful technique to evaluate the cause of acute dyspnea in the emergency setting is lung ultrasound, which can distinguish pulmonary edema from an AECOPD. The bedside recognition of diffuse sonographic vertical artifacts called comet tail or B lines suggests the presence of pulmonary edema.[26]

The prevalence of pulmonary embolism in patients hospitalized with an AECOPD has been reported to be 25%.[27] Notably, this study excluded those with antecedent signs of infection, so was limited to unexplained AECOPD.[28] These patients more frequently exhibit signs of cardiac failure and pleurisy. A higher vigilance for pulmonary embolism and testing with computed tomography angiography should be considered in this group.

Box 1
Initial studies for confirmed or suspected cases of the acute exacerbation of chronic obstructive pulmonary disease

Complete blood count and differential

Complete metabolic panel

Arterial blood gas

Brain natriuretic peptide

Baseline electrocardiogram

Chest radiograph (two-view, posteroanterior and lateral)

Inpatient spirometry confirming a diagnosis of COPD in patients who have never had spirometry (or prior spirometry records are unattainable)

Evaluation for pulmonary embolism in unexplained exacerbations

Lung ultrasound by trained providers may be considered

Finally, misdiagnosis of COPD has been reported to exceed 25%[29] and is a result of underuse of spirometry in the primary care setting. Therefore, for patients who have never had spirometry (or for whom records are not attainable), inpatient spirometry once clinically stabilized may be performed unless contraindications exist.

EMERGENCY ROOM MANAGEMENT AND TRIAGING
Emergency Room Management

Patients presenting to the emergency room should be rapidly assessed for the presence of acute respiratory failure and stabilized.[1,23] Patients suspected of having an AECOPD should receive nebulized short-acting bronchodilator and supplemental oxygen if required to maintain a saturation of 88% to 92%. Higher levels should be avoided because hyperoxia has been associated with worsening respiratory acidosis.[22,30] In a randomized controlled trial of titrated oxygen therapy (maintaining saturations between 88% and 92%) or nontitrated high-flow oxygen via facemask in prehospital care for COPD exacerbations, titrated oxygen therapy resulted in a 78% reduction in mortality and improved respiratory acidosis and hypercapnia.[31]

A comprehensive evaluation for alternate causes of respiratory decompensation should be completed. The medical management of patients confirmed to have an AECOPD is outlined in the following section; hospitalized patients should receive short courses of corticosteroids, and antibiotics therapy is contingent on the presence of increased sputum purulence.[1,23] Patients with acute respiratory acidosis should be stabilized with noninvasive positive pressure ventilation, (NIPPV) unless contraindications exist.

Criteria for Triaging

Listed next are recommended criteria for admission to a medical ward and respiratory or medical intensive care unit, adapted from guidelines from the GOLD committee.

Proposed criteria for admission to a respiratory or medical intensive care unit:

- Altered mental status
- Need for invasive or noninvasive mechanical ventilation
- Hypoxemia refractory to supplemental oxygen where the fraction of inspired oxygen exceeds 40%
- Presence of other conditions requiring intensive care unit admission

Proposed criteria for admission to the general medical ward (as opposed to home discharge):

- Failure of symptoms to resolve with nebulizer and steroids alone
- New or worsening oxygen requirement
- New or worsening hypercapnia (as evidenced by $Paco_2$ >10 mm Hg greater than baseline or pH <7.35)
- Concomitant acute congestive heart failure or pneumonia
- New or worsening renal or liver impairment
- Inadequate outpatient support

Hospital at home based programs can be considered for stable patients without respiratory failure.[23] A meta-analysis of eight trials found that selected patients could be safely managed at home with lower readmission rates and a trend to lower mortality.[32] There was insufficient evidence to conclude on the effect on quality of life, hospital-acquired infections, and costs. Careful patient selection is required; altered mental status, acute changes on chest radiograph or electrocardiogram, respiratory acidosis, or other exacerbated comorbidities were exclusion criteria.

Assessing Disease Severity

The most commonly used scoring system for assessing the severity of a COPD exacerbation is the dyspnea, eosinopenia, consolidation, acidemia, and fibrillation (DECAF) score, which predicts the risk of in-hospital mortality.[33]

Of note, patients using long-term oxygen therapy (LTOT) or who otherwise had other comorbidities resulting in a life expectancy of less than 12 months were excluded. Although it has undergone rigorous validation in the United Kingdom, implementation is not recommended by international consensus guidelines. The score is useful in monitoring patients who have high-risk scores; those admitted to a medical ward should be closely monitored with a low threshold for escalation in care.

INPATIENT MANAGEMENT
Antibiotics

For the subset of COPD exacerbations with increased cough and sputum purulence, antibiotics have been shown to reduce the risk of short-term mortality by 77%, decrease the risk of treatment failure by 53%, with a small increase in the risk of diarrhea.[34] However, the benefit is less clear when including trials that did not require purulent sputum as an inclusion criteria; a recent meta-analysis found no effect on mortality, treatment failure, or length of stay on inpatients not admitted to an intensive care unit.[35]

Therefore, antibiotic therapy is recommended for the following patients[1]:

- Those with all three of the following:
  ○ Increased sputum volume
  ○ Sputum purulence
  ○ Dyspnea

Or

- Those with two signs including sputum purulence or
- If mechanical ventilation is required

The duration of antibiotics should not exceed 5 to 7 days and oral antibiotics are preferred.

Biomarkers for active pulmonary bacterial infection are an area of active research. Point-of-care testing of C-reactive protein may be a way to reduce unnecessary use of antibiotics without harming patients who have an AECOPD. Studies suggest that antibiotics are most beneficial when the C-reactive protein level is greater than or equal to 40 mg/L.[36,37]

Similarly, treatment guided by procalcitonin, a sensitive biomarker of bacterial infection, has been studied in hospitalized patients with AECOPD.[38] Procalcitonin-guided therapy was poorly adopted by providers and was not associated with a decrease in total antibiotic days provided; however, a low procalcitonin level was associated with a 25.5% decrease in intravenous antibiotics, suggesting increased comfort stepping down from intravenous to oral therapy.[38]

Sputum cultures are not required unless patients display evidence of pneumonia; require invasive mechanical ventilation; have severe airflow obstruction; or have frequent exacerbations with antibiotic use, which increases the risk of resistant organisms.

Corticosteroid Therapy

Systemic corticosteroids are recommended for all patients hospitalized for an AECOPD.[1,23] A meta-analysis demonstrated that compared with placebo, systemic corticosteroids reduced the risk of treatment failure and length of stay while improving FEV_1; however, adverse events were common, occurring in one in six people treated.[39] There is no difference in outcomes when comparing oral versus parental treatment or longer versus shorter duration.[40] Therefore, for patients admitted to a general ward, an oral dose of 40 mg daily or steroid equivalent for 5 days is preferred unless contraindication to oral feeding exists. Since the implementation of shorter courses of steroids in 2014, there has been a significant decrease in pneumonia admissions and all-cause mortality, although the causal nature of this relationship is not established.[41]

There is evidence that blood eosinophil levels may be used to guide treatment with corticosteroids; a randomized controlled trial found that patients treated with eosinophil-guided therapy were less likely to receive corticosteroids and there was no significant difference in quality of life.[42] Patients with low eosinophil counts had greater treatment failure rates with prednisone therapy. More studies are needed to determine the safety of eosinophil-guided therapy.

Noninvasive Positive Pressure Ventilation

NIPPV is the first-line mode of ventilatory support in patients with acute hypercapnic respiratory failure. It reduces the need for invasive mechanical ventilation, hospital length of stay, and mortality.[43–46]

The following are indications for NIPPV[1]:

- Tachypnea or increased work of breathing despite treatment with supplemental oxygen and nebulized bronchodilators
- Acute respiratory acidosis on blood gas analysis (pH <7.35; $Paco_2$ >45 mm Hg)
- Mild alteration in mental status, which is attributed solely to hypercapnia

Contraindications to NIPPV include:

- Hemodynamic instability or cardiopulmonary arrest
- Altered mental status not attributable to hypercapnia alone
- Poor secretion clearance, hemoptysis, active vomiting, upper gastrointestinal bleeding, or other airway compromise
- Recent facial surgery or trauma

Patients who fail NIPPV and are ultimately intubated have higher mortality compared with patients who underwent endotracheal intubation without an NIPPV trial.[47] Therefore, careful patient selection and monitoring is recommended.

More research is needed in determining the optimal mode of delivery of NIPPV because there was significant heterogeneity across the trials. NIPPV is safely discontinued without weaning after 4 hours of stable unassisted breathing.[48]

CONSEQUENCES OF CHRONIC OBSTRUCTIVE PULMONARY DISEASE EXACERBATIONS
Recovery

Patients usually recover their lung function within a median time of 7 days.[21] Recovery of lung function is related to the magnitude of the decrease in lung function and the severity of symptoms at the onset of exacerbation. Return to baseline peak flow is complete in only 75% of exacerbations at Day 35 and in some cases lung function and symptoms may not recover to baseline values at 3 months.[21] Longer symptom duration has been linked to poor health status and a shorter time until the next exacerbation.[49]

Prognosis

The risk of readmission has been reported as 60%[50] and the risk of death 23% in the year following a hospitalization for AECOPD.[51] Long-term use of oral corticosteroids, higher $Paco_2$, and older age were identified as risk factors associated with higher mortality.[51]

PREVENTATIVE STRATEGIES

Discharge care bundles have been studied as a means to ensure the delivery of optimal care.[23] Clinical trials have shown mixed results because significant heterogeneity exists in the components of the bundled intervention.[52] Therefore, although implementation of interventions known to reduce exacerbations is recommended, their combined effectiveness in the form of distinct bundles remains an active area of study. Outlined in **Table 1** and discussed next are interventions known to reduce the risk of future exacerbations.

Pharmacologic Therapy

Initial inhaler therapy

Long-acting bronchodilator therapy is recommended by all expert groups for the prevention of COPD exacerbations,[1,53,54] and should be prescribed on discharge.

For patients who have not been on therapy beforehand, initiation of a long-acting muscarinic agent (LAMA) is recommended. Previous studies have shown increased efficacy in LAMAs in reducing exacerbations compared with long-acting β-agonists (LABAs).[55,56]

For patients who are highly symptomatic at baseline, initial therapy with combined LAMA/LABA has been shown to improve dyspnea relative to LAMA monotherapy, with an unclear benefit on exacerbations.[57] Consequently, LAMA/LABA therapy may be considered as first-line.

Inhaled corticosteroids are beneficial for patients with COPD who have a history of asthma or atopy, peripheral eosinophilia, or frequent exacerbations.[1] For hospitalized patients who have peripheral eosinophilia (absolute eosinophilic count exceeding

Table 1 Preventive strategies to reduce the frequency of AECOPD	
Category	**Intervention**
Pharmacologic therapy	Long-acting bronchodilators Inhaled corticosteroids Macrolide therapy Phosphodiesterase-4 inhibitor
Nonpharmacologic therapy	Smoking cessation Influenza and pneumococcal vaccination Supplemental oxygen Pulmonary rehabilitation Noninvasive positive pressure ventilation Self-management Palliative care

100 cells/µL), initial therapy with combined LABA/inhaled corticosteroid may be considered. However, inhaled corticosteroid is associated with pneumonia.[58]

Dose escalation

Dose escalation according to the GOLD guidelines is provided in **Fig. 2**. For patients previously on maximal inhaler therapy before admission, addition of a standing macrolide or phosphodiesterase-4 inhibitor should be considered. The use of long-term oral corticosteroid is no longer recommended in patients with COPD, and has been associated with increased mortality.[59]

Macrolide therapy

Azithromycin has been shown to decrease exacerbations in patients with frequent exacerbations.[60] The greatest benefit was seen in those with better lung function, and in those who were not current smokers.[61] Maintenance azithromycin treatment is

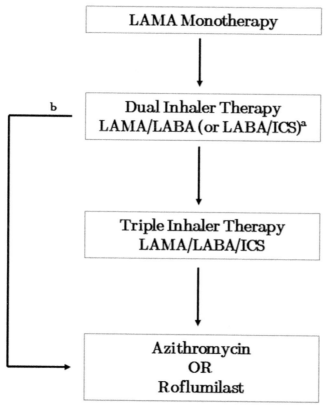

Fig. 2. Dose escalation of inhaler therapy after an exacerbation of chronic obstructive pulmonary disease. ICS, inhaled corticosteroid. [a] LABA/ICS is considered in patients with elevated peripheral eosinophil counts (>100 cells/µL). [b] In patients with low peripheral eosinophil counts (<100 cells/µL), escalation from LAMA/LABA with addition of azithromycin or roflumilast should be considered. (*Adapted from* Global Strategy for the Diagnosis, Management, and Prevention of Chronic Obstructive Pulmonary Disease 2020 Report. Global Initiative for Chronic Obstructive Lung Disease (GOLD). Available at: https://goldcopd.org/wp-content/uploads/2019/11/GOLD-2020-REPORT-ver1.0wms.pdf. Accessed Feb 7 2020; with permission.)

associated with a small increase in hearing loss[60]; however, long-term side effects, such as cardiovascular events and bacterial resistance, are unknown.

Phosphodiesterase inhibition

Roflumilast is a phosphodiesterase-4 inhibitor that reduces airway inflammation and has been shown to reduce exacerbations and improve lung function in patients with an FEV_1 less than 50% and history of chronic bronchitis.[62,63] Side effects include weight loss and diarrhea, and caution should be used in patients with depression or suicidality.

Smoking Cessation

Smoking cessation is one of the most cost-effective interventions in the management of COPD and reduces symptom burden, mortality, exacerbation rates, and lung function decline.[53,64] A combination of pharmacologic interventions and behavioral strategies is recommended. A meta-analysis of smoking cessation interventions found that any counseling resulted in a modest increase in smoking cessation. There was no additional benefit in higher intensity versus lower intensity counseling.[65]

Vaccines

Influenza vaccination has been shown to reduce COPD exacerbations on meta-analysis of 11 studies.[66] The role of pneumococcal vaccination in reducing exacerbations has not been clearly demonstrated. There was no benefit of pneumococcal vaccination on pneumonia incidence, acute exacerbations, hospital admissions, or emergency department visits on meta-analysis.[67] However, combining both influenza vaccines resulted in fewer exacerbations related to respiratory infections,[68] and both vaccinations are recommended.

Oxygen

LTOT is indicated in patients with:

- Resting hypoxemia (PaO_2 <55 mm Hg or oxygen saturation <89%), or
- PaO_2 between 55 and 60 mm Hg with cor pulmonale and erythrocytosis (hematocrit >50%)

LTOT in this population has been shown to reduce mortality in COPD.[69,70] There was no additional benefit in prescribing LTOT to patients with mild to moderate exertional hypoxemia (ie, with resting saturation between 89% and 93%, and moderate desaturation to 80% with exertion).[71] If patients are prescribed oxygen on discharge after an AECOPD, continued need should be evaluated in 60 to 90 days.

Pulmonary Rehabilitation

Pulmonary rehabilitation is a comprehensive program of supervised exercise training and behavioral therapy, including breathing exercises, smoking cessation counseling, and self-management. It has been shown to reduce hospital readmissions by 66% if initiated within 3 weeks of discharge.[1] It is associated with improved health-related quality of life and exercise capacity.

The maximal benefit has been seen in trials where the intervention is initiated in the postexacerbation period.[72] A randomized controlled trial showed an increase toward 1-year mortality when pulmonary rehabilitation was initiated as an inpatient compared with usual care,[73] perhaps a result of underuse of posthospital pulmonary rehabilitation. Home-based programs have shown similar efficacy to center-based programs,[74,75] and is a reasonable alternative if there is limited access to outpatient structured programs.

Noninvasive Positive Pressure Ventilation

NIPPV has been shown to reduce rehospitalizations among patients with an AECOPD.[76] A landmark trial compared home NIPPV with oxygen to oxygen therapy alone in patients with hypercapnia 2 to 4 weeks postdischarge and found a 17% reduction in the composite end point of readmission or death.[77] Higher pressures were targeted, with median inspiratory positive airway pressure of 24 and expiratory positive airway pressure of 4, and backup rate of 14, which is considered a high-intensity approach. Prior studies showing no benefit of NIPPV did not confirm the chronicity of hypercapnia or used a low-pressure approach. Therefore, assessing patients who had acute hypercapnia 2 to 4 weeks after discharge and initiating NIPPV with a moderate to high pressure is recommended.

Self-Management Strategies

Self-management strategies empower patients to adapt behaviors and skills to manage their COPD, reduces respiratory-related exacerbations, and improves exercise performance and disease literacy.[78] Important self-management domains in the periexacerbation period include: ensuring compliance with therapy, smoking cessation, vaccination, physical activity and exercise training, and pulmonary rehabilitation.[79] Avoiding stimuli for recurrent exacerbations and awareness of declining symptoms should be highlighted.

Palliative Care

Despite high symptom burden, palliative care remains underused in patients with severe COPD.[80] Early palliative counseling for highly symptomatic patients, independent of prognosis, has been shown to be beneficial when the following themes were addressed[81]:

- Emotional symptoms
- Respiratory symptoms
- Illness understanding
- Prognostic awareness
- Coping with COPD

In addition, advanced care planning and establishing patients' preferences regarding end-of-life care in the event of further clinical deterioration is prudent.

Hospice referral is appropriate in patients with advanced COPD and limited life expectancy. Patients with advanced COPD without significant life-limiting comorbidities should undergo a thorough outpatient prognostic assessment; pulmonary rehabilitation and consideration of advanced therapies beyond the scope of this article, including lung transplantation or lung volume reduction surgery, should be discussed before hospice referral.

SUMMARY

An AECOPD requiring hospitalization significantly increases the risk of subsequent rehospitalization and death. Equal emphasis should be placed on reducing this risk of future decompensation. NIPPV has dramatically improved outcomes in patients with acute hypercapnic respiratory failure. However, the chronicity of hypercapnia should be demonstrated before continuing NIPPV in the outpatient setting. Although structured care bundles have not been shown to be efficacious, individual components of smoking cessation, early referral to pulmonary rehabilitation, optimal inhaler therapy, advanced oral therapies including chronic antibiotic or phosphodiesterase therapy, and vaccinations improve outcomes in patients with COPD. Lastly, because breathlessness is one of the most distressing symptoms a human can experience it is equally important to provide palliation. Despite the poor prognosis of AECOPD, patients are empowered through self-management programs in their battle against this lethal disease.

REFERENCES

1. Global Strategy for the Diagnosis, Management, and Prevention of Chronic Obstructive Pulmonary Disease. Global Initiative for Chronic Obstructive Lung Disease. 2020. Available at: https://goldcopd.org/wp-content/uploads/2019/11/GOLD-2020-REPORT-ver1.0wms.pdf. Accessed February 7, 2020.
2. Ford ES, Croft JB, Mannino DM, et al. COPD surveillance–United States, 1999-2011. Chest 2013;144:284–305.
3. Vos T, Flaxman AD, Naghavi M, et al. Years lived with disability (YLDs) for 1160 sequelae of 289 diseases and injuries 1990-2010: a systematic analysis for the Global Burden of Disease Study 2010. Lancet 2012;380:2163–96.
4. Lozano R, Naghavi M, Foreman K, et al. Global and regional mortality from 235 causes of death for 20 age groups in 1990 and 2010: a systematic analysis for the Global Burden of Disease Study 2010. Lancet 2012;380:2095–128.
5. Hurst JR, Vestbo J, Anzueto A, et al. Susceptibility to exacerbation in chronic obstructive pulmonary disease. N Engl J Med 2010;363:1128–38.
6. Mahler DA, Wells CK. Evaluation of clinical methods for rating dyspnea. Chest 1988;93:580–6.
7. Jones PW, Harding G, Berry P, et al. Development and first validation of the COPD assessment test. Eur Respir J 2009;34:648–54.
8. Jafarinejad H, Moghoofei M, Mostafaei S, et al. Worldwide prevalence of viral infection in AECOPD patients: a meta-analysis. Microb pathogenesis 2017;113:190–6.
9. Greenberg SB, Allen M, Wilson J, et al. Respiratory viral infections in adults with and without chronic obstructive pulmonary disease. Am J Respir Crit Care Med 2000;162:167–73.
10. Wark PA, Tooze M, Powell H, et al. Viral and bacterial infection in acute asthma and chronic obstructive pulmonary disease increases the risk of readmission. Respirology 2013;18:996–1002.
11. McManus TE, Marley AM, Baxter N, et al. Respiratory viral infection in exacerbations of COPD. Respir Med 2008;102:1575–80.
12. Wang H, Anthony D, Selemidis S, et al. Resolving viral-induced secondary bacterial infection in COPD: a concise review. Front Immunol 2018;9:2345.
13. Monso E, Ruiz J, Rosell A, et al. Bacterial infection in chronic obstructive pulmonary disease. A study of stable and exacerbated outpatients using the protected specimen brush. Am J Respir Crit Care Med 1995;152:1316–20.
14. Pela R, Marchesani F, Agostinelli C, et al. Airways microbial flora in COPD patients in stable clinical conditions and during exacerbations: a bronchoscopic investigation. Monaldi Arch Chest Dis 1998;53:262–7.
15. Sethi S, Muscarella K, Evans N, et al. Airway inflammation and etiology of acute exacerbations of chronic bronchitis. Chest 2000;118:1557–65.

16. Sethi S, Murphy TF. Bacterial infection in chronic obstructive pulmonary disease in 2000: a state-of-the-art review. Clin Microbiol Rev 2001;14:336–63.

17. Wilkinson TMA, Aris E, Bourne S, et al. A prospective, observational cohort study of the seasonal dynamics of airway pathogens in the aetiology of exacerbations in COPD. Thorax 2017;72:919–27.

18. Qiu H, Tan K, Long F, et al. The Burden of COPD Morbidity Attributable to the Interaction between Ambient air pollution and Temperature in Chengdu, China. Int J Environ Res Public Health 2018;15.

19. Larkin A, Hystad P. Towards personal exposures: how technology is changing air pollution and health research. Curr Environ Health Rep 2017;4:463–71.

20. Anthonisen NR, Manfreda J, Warren CP, et al. Antibiotic therapy in exacerbations of chronic obstructive pulmonary disease. Ann Intern Med 1987;106:196–204.

21. Seemungal TA, Donaldson GC, Bhowmik A, et al. Time course and recovery of exacerbations in patients with chronic obstructive pulmonary disease. Am J Respir Crit Care Med 2000;161:1608–13.

22. Brill SE, Wedzicha JA. Oxygen therapy in acute exacerbations of chronic obstructive pulmonary disease. Int J Chron Obstruct Pulmon Dis 2014;9: 1241–52.

23. Wedzicha JAEC-C, Miravitlles M, Hurst JR, et al. Management of COPD exacerbations: a European respiratory Society/American Thoracic Society guideline. Eur Respir J 2017;49.

24. Snow V, Lascher S, Mottur-Pilson C. Evidence base for management of acute exacerbations of chronic obstructive pulmonary disease. Ann Intern Med 2001;134: 595–9.

25. Emerman CL, Cydulka RK. Evaluation of high-yield criteria for chest radiography in acute exacerbation of chronic obstructive pulmonary disease. Ann Emerg Med 1993;22:680–4.

26. Volpicelli G, Cardinale L, Garofalo G, et al. Usefulness of lung ultrasound in the bedside distinction between pulmonary edema and exacerbation of COPD. Emerg Radiol 2008;15:145–51.

27. Tillie-Leblond I, Marquette CH, Perez T, et al. Pulmonary embolism in patients with unexplained exacerbation of chronic obstructive pulmonary disease: prevalence and risk factors. Ann Intern Med 2006;144:390–6.

28. Aleva FE, Voets L, Simons SO, et al. Prevalence and localization of pulmonary embolism in unexplained acute exacerbations of COPD: a systematic review and meta-analysis. Chest 2017;151:544–54.

29. Jain VV, Allison DR, Andrews S, et al. Misdiagnosis among frequent exacerbators of clinically diagnosed asthma and COPD in absence of confirmation of airflow obstruction. Lung 2015;193:505–12.

30. Abdo WF, Heunks LM. Oxygen-induced hypercapnia in COPD: myths and facts. Crit Care 2012;16:323.

31. Austin MA, Wills KE, Blizzard L, et al. Effect of high flow oxygen on mortality in chronic obstructive pulmonary disease patients in prehospital setting: randomised controlled trial. BMJ 2010;341:c5462.

32. Jeppesen E, Brurberg KG, Vist GE, et al. Hospital at home for acute exacerbations of chronic obstructive pulmonary disease. Cochrane Database Syst Rev 2012:CD003573.

33. Steer J, Gibson J, Bourke SC. The DECAF score: predicting hospital mortality in exacerbations of chronic obstructive pulmonary disease. Thorax 2012;67:970–6.

34. Ram FS, Rodriguez-Roisin R, Granados-Navarrete A, et al. Antibiotics for exacerbations of chronic obstructive pulmonary disease. Cochrane Database Syst Rev 2006:CD004403.

35. Vollenweider DJ, Frei A, Steurer-Stey CA, et al. Antibiotics for exacerbations of chronic obstructive pulmonary disease. Cochrane Database Syst Rev 2018;(10):CD010257.

36. Llor C, Moragas A, Hernandez S, et al. Efficacy of antibiotic therapy for acute exacerbations of mild to moderate chronic obstructive pulmonary disease. Am J Respir Crit Care Med 2012;186:716–23.

37. Miravitlles M, Moragas A, Hernandez S, et al. Is it possible to identify exacerbations of mild to moderate COPD that do not require antibiotic treatment? Chest 2013;144:1571–7.

38. Ulrich RJ, McClung D, Wang BR, et al. Introduction of procalcitonin testing and antibiotic utilization for acute exacerbations of chronic obstructive pulmonary disease. Infect Dis 2019;12. 1178633719852626.

39. Walters JA, Tan DJ, White CJ, et al. Systemic corticosteroids for acute exacerbations of chronic obstructive pulmonary disease. Cochrane Database Syst Rev 2014:CD001288.

40. Leuppi JD, Schuetz P, Bingisser R, et al. Short-term vs conventional glucocorticoid therapy in acute exacerbations of chronic obstructive pulmonary disease: the REDUCE randomized clinical trial. JAMA 2013;309:2223–31.

41. Sivapalan P, Ingebrigtsen TS, Rasmussen DB, et al. COPD exacerbations: the impact of long versus short courses of oral corticosteroids on mortality and pneumonia: nationwide data on 67 000 patients with COPD followed for 12 months. BMJ Open Respir Res 2019;6:e000407.

42. Bafadhel M, McKenna S, Terry S, et al. Blood eosinophils to direct corticosteroid treatment of exacerbations of chronic obstructive pulmonary disease: a randomized placebo-controlled trial. Am J Respir Crit Care Med 2012;186:48–55.

43. Brochard L, Mancebo J, Wysocki M, et al. Noninvasive ventilation for acute exacerbations of chronic obstructive pulmonary disease. N Engl J Med 1995;333:817–22.

44. Kramer N, Meyer TJ, Meharg J, et al. Randomized, prospective trial of noninvasive positive pressure ventilation in acute respiratory failure. Am J Respir Crit Care Med 1995;151:1799–806.

45. Plant PK, Owen JL, Elliott MW. Early use of non-invasive ventilation for acute exacerbations of chronic obstructive pulmonary disease on general respiratory wards: a multicentre randomised controlled trial. Lancet 2000;355:1931–5.

46. Lindenauer PK, Stefan MS, Shieh MS, et al. Outcomes associated with invasive and noninvasive ventilation among patients hospitalized with exacerbations of chronic obstructive pulmonary disease. JAMA Intern Med 2014;174:1982–93.

47. Mehta AB, Douglas IS, Walkey AJ. Hospital noninvasive ventilation case volume and outcomes of acute exacerbations of chronic obstructive pulmonary disease. Ann Am Thorac Soc 2016;13:1752–9.

48. Sellares J, Ferrer M, Anton A, et al. Discontinuing noninvasive ventilation in severe chronic obstructive pulmonary disease exacerbations: a randomised controlled trial. Eur Respir J 2017;50.

49. Donaldson GC, Law M, Kowlessar B, et al. Impact of prolonged exacerbation recovery in chronic obstructive pulmonary disease. Am J Respir Crit Care Med 2015;192:943–50.

50. Garcia-Aymerich J, Farrero E, Felez MA, et al. Risk factors of readmission to hospital for a COPD exacerbation: a prospective study. Thorax 2003;58:100–5.

51. Groenewegen KH, Schols AM, Wouters EF. Mortality and mortality-related factors after hospitalization for acute exacerbation of COPD. Chest 2003;124:459–67.

52. Ospina MB, Mrklas K, Deuchar L, et al. A systematic review of the effectiveness of discharge care bundles for patients with COPD. Thorax 2017;72:31–9.

53. Wedzicha JA, Calverley PMA, Albert RK, et al. Prevention of COPD exacerbations: a European respiratory Society/American Thoracic Society guideline. Eur Respir J 2017;50.

54. Criner GJ, Bourbeau J, Diekemper RL, et al. Prevention of acute exacerbations of COPD: American College of chest Physicians and Canadian Thoracic Society guideline. Chest 2015;147:894–942.

55. Vogelmeier C, Hederer B, Glaab T, et al. Tiotropium versus salmeterol for the prevention of exacerbations of COPD. N Engl J Med 2011;364:1093–103.

56. Decramer ML, Chapman KR, Dahl R, et al. Once-daily indacaterol versus tiotropium for patients with severe chronic obstructive pulmonary disease (INVIGORATE): a randomised, blinded, parallel-group study. Lancet Respir Med 2013;1: 524–33.

57. Mahler DA, Kerwin E, Ayers T, et al. FLIGHT1 and FLIGHT2: efficacy and safety of QVA149 (Indacaterol/Glycopyrrolate) versus its monocomponents and placebo in patients with chronic obstructive pulmonary disease. Am J Respir Crit Care Med 2015;192:1068–79.

58. Kew KM, Seniukovich A. Inhaled steroids and risk of pneumonia for chronic obstructive pulmonary disease. Cochrane Database Syst Rev 2014:CD010115.

59. Horita N, Miyazawa N, Morita S, et al. Evidence suggesting that oral corticosteroids increase mortality in stable chronic obstructive pulmonary disease. Respir Res 2014;15:37.

60. Albert RK, Connett J, Bailey WC, et al. Azithromycin for prevention of exacerbations of COPD. N Engl J Med 2011;365:689–98.

61. Han MK, Tayob N, Murray S, et al. Predictors of chronic obstructive pulmonary disease exacerbation reduction in response to daily azithromycin therapy. Am J Respir Crit Care Med 2014;189:1503–8.

62. Fabbri LM, Calverley PM, Izquierdo-Alonso JL, et al. Roflumilast in moderate-to-severe chronic obstructive pulmonary disease treated with longacting bronchodilators: two randomised clinical trials. Lancet 2009;374:695–703.

63. Martinez FJ, Calverley PM, Goehring UM, et al. Effect of roflumilast on exacerbations in patients with severe chronic obstructive pulmonary disease uncontrolled by combination therapy (REACT): a multicentre randomised controlled trial. Lancet 2015;385:857–66.

64. Hersh CP, DeMeo DL, Al-Ansari E, et al. Predictors of survival in severe, early onset COPD. Chest 2004;126:1443–51.

65. Stead LF, Bergson G, Lancaster T. Physician advice for smoking cessation. Cochrane Database Syst Rev 2008:CD000165.

66. Kopsaftis Z, Wood-Baker R, Poole P. Influenza vaccine for chronic obstructive pulmonary disease (COPD). Cochrane Database Syst Rev 2018;(6):CD002733.

67. Walters JA, Smith S, Poole P, et al. Injectable vaccines for preventing pneumococcal infection in patients with chronic obstructive pulmonary disease. Cochrane Database Syst Rev 2010:CD001390.

68. Furumoto A, Ohkusa Y, Chen M, et al. Additive effect of pneumococcal vaccine and influenza vaccine on acute exacerbation in patients with chronic lung disease. Vaccine 2008;26:4284–9.

69. Continuous or nocturnal oxygen therapy in hypoxemic chronic obstructive lung disease: a clinical trial. Nocturnal Oxygen Therapy Trial Group. Ann Intern Med 1980;93:391–8.
70. Long term domiciliary oxygen therapy in chronic hypoxic cor pulmonale complicating chronic bronchitis and emphysema. Report of the Medical Research Council Working Party. Lancet 1981;1:681–6.
71. Albert RK, Au DH, Blackford AL, et al. A randomized trial of long-term oxygen for COPD with moderate desaturation. N Engl J Med 2016;375:1617–27.
72. Ibrahim W, Harvey-Dunstan TC, Greening NJ. Rehabilitation in chronic respiratory diseases: in-hospital and post-exacerbation pulmonary rehabilitation. Respirology 2019.
73. Greening NJ, Williams JE, Hussain SF, et al. An early rehabilitation intervention to enhance recovery during hospital admission for an exacerbation of chronic respiratory disease: randomised controlled trial. BMJ 2014;349:g4315.
74. Vasilopoulou M, Papaioannou AI, Kaltsakas G, et al. Home-based maintenance tele-rehabilitation reduces the risk for acute exacerbations of COPD, hospitalisations and emergency department visits. Eur Respir J 2017;49.
75. Bhatt SP, Patel SB, Anderson EM, et al. Video telehealth pulmonary rehabilitation intervention in COPD reduces 30-day readmissions. Am J Respir Crit Care Med 2019.
76. Kohnlein T, Windisch W, Kohler D, et al. Non-invasive positive pressure ventilation for the treatment of severe stable chronic obstructive pulmonary disease: a prospective, multicentre, randomised, controlled clinical trial. Lancet Respir Med 2014;2:698–705.
77. Murphy PB, Rehal S, Arbane G, et al. Effect of home noninvasive ventilation with oxygen therapy vs oxygen therapy alone on hospital readmission or death after an acute COPD exacerbation: a randomized clinical trial. JAMA 2017;317:2177–86.
78. Lenferink A, Brusse-Keizer M, van der Valk PD, et al. Self-management interventions including action plans for exacerbations versus usual care in patients with chronic obstructive pulmonary disease. Cochrane Database Syst Rev 2017;(8):CD011682.
79. Effing TW, Vercoulen JH, Bourbeau J, et al. Definition of a COPD self-management intervention: International Expert group consensus. Eur Respir J 2016;48:46–54.
80. Maddocks M, Lovell N, Booth S, et al. Palliative care and management of troublesome symptoms for people with chronic obstructive pulmonary disease. Lancet 2017;390:988–1002.
81. Iyer AS, Dionne-Odom JN, Ford SM, et al. A formative evaluation of patient and family caregiver perspectives on early palliative care in chronic obstructive pulmonary disease across disease severity. Ann Am Thorac Soc 2019;16:1024–33.

Treatment of Acute Venous Thromboembolism

Sashi Nair, MD[a], Nina Garza, DO, MPH[a], Matt George, MD[b], Scott Kaatz, DO, MSc[c],*

KEYWORDS

- Deep vein thrombosis • Pulmonary embolism • Anticoagulation • Thrombolytic
- Risk stratification

KEY POINTS

- Guidelines suggest using direct oral anticoagulants (DOAC) over traditional therapy for low-molecular-weight heparin (LMWH) and warfarin for acute deep vein thrombosis (DVT) and pulmonary embolism (PE) based on their safety profile.
- The best route, dose, or need for thrombolytic treatment of intermediate-risk PE is an active area of research, and a definitive therapeutic approach is not currently established.
- Guidelines suggest against the routine use of thrombolytics in most patients with DVT.
- The use of DOACs in patients with cancer-associated DVT and PE is emerging, and guidance is beginning to suggest their use instead of LMWH as first-line treatment.

INTRODUCTION AND EPIDEMIOLOGY

Acute venous thromboembolism (VTE) has an annual incidence rate of 1 to 2 per 1000 persons in the United States.[1] Despite increasing efforts to prevent occurrence, rates continue to increase in hospitalized patients across the United States.[2] VTE also represents a significant source of health care expenditures—with cost estimated between $14 billion and 27 billion annually.[3] This article reviews the current evidence regarding treatment of deep vein thrombosis (DVT) and pulmonary embolism (PE), as well as review updates in special populations (cancer, obesity, and renal disease).

PULMONARY EMBOLISM
Risk Stratification

PE has a wide spectrum of presentations and outcomes ranging from incidental imaging findings to cardiovascular collapse, thus risk stratification of PE is essential.

Patients who are hemodynamically unstable (traditionally defined as a persistent systolic blood pressure less than 90 mm/hg or requirement of vasopressors, with

[a] Department of Medicine, Henry Ford Hospital, 2799 West Grand Boulevard, Detroit, MI 48202, USA; [b] Division of Hospital Medicine, Henry Ford West Bloomfield Hospital, 6777 West Maple Road, West Bloomfield, MI 48322, USA; [c] Division of Hospital Medicine, Henry Ford Hospital, 2799 West Grand Boulevard, Detroit, MI 48202, USA
* Corresponding author.
E-mail address: Skaatz1@hfhs.org

Med Clin N Am 104 (2020) 631–646
https://doi.org/10.1016/j.mcna.2020.03.004
0025-7125/20/© 2020 Elsevier Inc. All rights reserved.
medical.theclinics.com

clinical or biochemical signs of hypoperfusion) are defined as those with high-risk or massive PE.[4] Hemodynamically stable patients require further stratification. The Pulmonary Embolism Severity Index (PESI) score and the simplified (sPESI) score are risk assessment models that have been incorporated into guidelines.[5,6] Multiple online risk calculators and mobile applications are available to facilitate application of these scores. Patients who have an elevated risk based on PESI/sPESI are classified as intermediate risk. Intermediate risk patients are further stratified. Those with both right heart strain on imaging, and positive troponins are classified as intermediate-high risk, those with either right heart strain or troponins are intermediate low risk. Low risk patients are defined by a low PESI/sPESI score. Patients who would otherwise have been classified as low risk by sPESI or PESI, but are found to have evidence of right heart strain or troponin elevation are known to have increased mortality and should be treated as intermediate risk.[4,7]

High-risk/massive pulmonary embolism

Initial stabilization of the patient with acute high-risk PE is based on lessons from patients with acute right heart failure.[8,9] This may include an intravenous (IV) fluid bolus of no more than 500 cc, as excess preload on an overdistended ventricle may worsen shock. Vasopressors may be required to maintain systemic perfusion with norepinephrine or dobutamine (preferred). Supplemental oxygen progressing to low tidal volume, low peak pressure ventilation can be used to support oxygenation as patients with PE are particularly sensitive to increased intrathoracic pressure. Case series have demonstrated the role of venoarterial extracorporeal membrane oxygenation as a bridge to definitive therapy, which may entail thrombolysis, embolectomy, or catheter-directed methods.[10]

The cornerstone of management in high-risk or massive PE is reperfusion. Systemic thrombolysis improves mortality in patients with high-risk PE albeit with an increased incidence of major bleeding and approximately 2% rate of intracranial hemorrhage (ICH).[11] In patients who have absolute contraindications to thrombolysis, surgical thrombectomy is a viable alternative with similar mortality rates.[12] In patients who are not candidates for systemic thrombolysis or surgical embolectomy, or in patients with failed thrombolysis, catheter-based therapies (**Table 1**) can be considered.

Intermediate risk/submassive pulmonary embolism

The role of thrombolysis in patients with intermediate-risk PE is not clear. The PEITHO trial randomized 1005 participants to receive placebo or weight-based (30–50 mg) tenecteplase in addition to standard of care. Results provided evidence that thrombolysis may decrease the combined endpoint of mortality or escalation of care at the cost of increased rate of ICH in patients with intermediate-risk PE.[18] There was no statistically significant difference in mortality, but there was a significant decrease in the rate of hemodynamic decompensation (1.6% vs 5%, odds ratio [OR] 0.3, $P = .002$). Thrombolytic treatment was associated with a significant increase in stroke (2.4% vs 0.2%, OR 12.1, $P = .003$) and extracranial bleed (6.3% vs 1.2%, OR 5.55, $P<.001$). Subsequent meta-analyses have yielded a significant mortality benefit in the intermediate-risk PE population and a signal toward less bleeding for patients younger than 65 years who receive thrombolysis compared with patients older than 65 years who receive thrombolysis.[19,20] However, the routine use of systemic thrombolysis in intermediate-high–risk patients has not been supported by either the European Society of Cardiology 2019 or American College of Chest Physicians 2016 guidelines.[4,21] Although available evidence for patients with intermediate-high–risk PE is unclear, patients should be closely monitored regardless of treatment choice,

Table 1
Catheter-based reperfusion strategies

Type	Principle	Selected Examples	Selected Studies
Catheter-directed lysis	Direct, local pulmonary arterial administration of thrombolytics can potentially reduce the required dose, increase efficacy, and improve safety	• Unifuse Catheter system • Cragg-McNamara system	• PERFECT[13]
Ultrasound-assisted thrombolysis	Local ultrasonic energy may facilitate penetration of thrombolysis into thrombi. Typically use slow infusion of 1-2 mg/min of tPA and 12-24-h dwell time of catheter in the pulmonary artery	• EKOSonic	• ULTIMA[14] • SEATTLE II[15]
Mechanical-assisted catheters	Use of mechanical disruption, suction, or rheolytic effects to disrupt thrombi can be used without thrombolysis in patients who have contraindications	• FlowTriever—mechanical disruption • Penumbra-indigo—rheolytic destruction • AngioVac-Suction thrombectomy	• FLARE[16] • EXTRACT-PE[17] (ongoing)

Unifuse Catheter system (AngioDynamics, Latham NY), Cragg-McNamara system (Medtronic, Minneapolis MN), EKOSonic (Boston Scientific, Marlborough MA), FlowTriever (Inari Medical, Irvine CA), Penumbra-indigo (Penumbra Inc, Alameda CA), AngioVac (AngioDynamics, Latham NY).
Abbreviation: tPA, tissue plasminogen activator.

as the median time to death or decompensation was 1.8 days in the placebo group in the PETHIOS trial.[18]

Controversy also exists regarding the dose of tissue plasminogen activator (tPA), with full dose considered to be 100 mg of alteplase given over 2 hours. The MOPPET trial enrolled 121 patients with "moderate" PE (determined by clot burden of greater than 70% involvement of thrombus in 2 or more lobar or the main pulmonary arteries) and randomized them to receive either 0.5 mg/kg (max 50 mg) or placebo in addition to standard of care. There was a statistically significant decrease in the rate of pulmonary hypertension and recurrent PE at 28 months (16% vs 63%, $P<.001$), as well as hospital length of stay (2.2 days vs 4.9 days, $P<.001$) but not in mortality (1.6% vs 5%, $P = .3$).[22]However, contrary evidence has emerged comparing full- versus reduced-dose tPA, showing no clear mortality or bleeding risk benefit with a reduced dose and demonstrating increased need for escalation of care.[23]

An alternative method of reduced-dose thrombolysis is intrapulmonary arterial administration with catheter-based therapies. Numerous devices are becoming available, consisting of an intrapulmonary catheter with or without the addition of energy-assisted thrombolysis or thrombectomy (see **Table 1**). Various studies have investigated these techniques; however, the role of catheter-based therapies for intermediate-high–risk PE is still unclear. Available evidence has shown favorable reductions in right ventricular size and pulmonary arterial pressure as surrogates for efficacy and mortality with minimal bleeding complications and rates of intracranial hemorrhage of less than 1%. To date no trials have demonstrated a mortality benefit.[13–17] Given the numerous therapeutic options and modalities available, many hospitals have built Pulmonary Embolism Response Teams (PERT) to provide management recommendations in these complex patients. The European Society of Cardiology has given a class IIa recommendation for consultation with a PERT team, although questions remain on optimal size, composition, and funding.[4]

There is no established role of thrombolysis or catheter-directed therapy for the intermediate-low–risk PE, hence the mainstay of therapy remains systemic anticoagulation.[4,21]

Low-risk pulmonary embolism

Patients with low-risk PE who have no other reason for hospitalization or additional barriers to treatment adherence can be managed at home with no increase immortality. The Outpatient Treatment of Pulmonary Embolism trial randomized 344 patients with low-risk PE to inpatient or outpatient treatment and demonstrated noninferiority of outpatient therapy.[24] The Hestia criteria have been developed to standardize the selection of these patients (**Box 1**).[25] If a patient lacks any of the Hestia criteria they may be an appropriate candidate for early discharge and home treatment.

Controversy still exists regarding the management of isolated small subsegmental PE. Interobserver variability can be as high as 50%, and in the absence of proximal DVT or risk factors, patients with isolated subsegmental PE who did not receive anticoagulation have a VTE recurrence rate and mortality similar to those who were anticoagulated.[26–28] Conservative management and close follow-up may be a reasonable treatment plan if there is no DVT.

DEEP VEIN THROMBOSIS
Distal Deep Vein Thrombosis

Anticoagulation for isolated distal calf vein thrombosis is controversial because the risk of PE is low; however, extention to the popliteal vein and hence a proximal DVT is of concern. The American College of Chest Physicians (ACCP) guidelines suggest either no anticoagulation plus mandatory Doppler surveillance for extention for more than 2 weeks or anticoagulation in patients with risk of extention.[21]

Box 1
The Hestia criteria for early discharge and home treatment of pulmonary embolism

- Hemodynamically unstable
- Thrombolysis or embolectomy needed
- Active bleeding or high risk for bleeding
- PE diagnosed while on anticoagulation
- Severe liver impairment
- Renal disease with creatinine clearance less than 30 mL/min
- Pregnancy
- Documented history of heparin-induced thrombocytopenia
- Supplemental oxygen required to maintain SaO_2 greater than 90% for more than 24 hours
- Severe pain needing IV pain medication required for more than 24 hours
- Medical or social reason for admission more than 24 hours

Adapted from Zondag W, Mos IC, Creemers-Schild D, et al. Outpatient treatment in patients with acute pulmonary embolism: the Hestia Study. J Thromb Haemost 2011;9(8):1501; with permission.

The CACTUS trial was reported after the publication of the ACCP guidelines and was terminated early because study drug expired and only half of the planned number of patients was enrolled. Two hundred fifty-nine outpatients with calf vein thrombosis and no history of cancer or previous DVT were randomized to low-molecular-weight heparin (LMWH) or placebo. There was no statistical difference in the composite outcome of extention to proximal veins, contralateral DVT, or PE, and there was more bleeding with LMWH versus placebo (4% vs 0%, 95% confidence interval 0.4–9.2).[29] This underpowered trial suggests more harm than benefit in treating low-risk, isolated calf vein thrombosis.

Catheter-Directed Thrombolysis for Acute Proximal Deep Vein Thrombosis

Thrombolysis, either systemic or catheter–based, using a variety of techniques has been shown to improve vein patency for treatment of DVT with the hope of decreasing postthrombotic syndrome. However, ACCP guidelines suggest anticoagulant therapy alone over catheter-directed thrombolysis.[21] A Cochrane systematic review of 1103 randomized patients in 17 trials found thrombolysis increased vein patency and reduced postthrombotic syndrome. However, this review did not include 692 patients in the ATTRACT trial.[30]

The ATTRACT trial randomized patients with acute proximal DVT to pharmacomechanical thrombolysis with tPA and thrombus aspiration or maceration with or without stenting plus anticoagulation versus anticoagulation alone with a primary outcome of postthrombotic syndrome between 6 and 24 months.[31] Pharmacomechanical thrombolysis showed no efficacy in the primary outcome (47% vs 48%), a trend in improvement in moderate-to-severe postthrombotic syndrome (18% vs 24%, $P = .04$ [<0.01 considered significant for multiple secondary outcomes]) and more major bleeding in the first 10 days (1.7% vs 0.3%, $P = .03$), but no difference in bleeding at 24-month follow-up. This trial indicates no long-term benefit and short-term harm with pharmacomechanical thrombolysis.

The ACCP guidelines suggest anticoagulation over thrombolysis for upper extremity DVT.[21] Candidates likely to benefit would have thrombus in most of the subclavian and axillary veins, symptoms of less than 14 days, good functional status, and low risk of bleeding.

Compression Stockings to Prevent Postthrombotic Syndrome

Postthrombotic syndrome can affect up to half of patients with proximal DVT, and use of compression stockings is thought to prevent venous dilatation and further valve damage. ACCP guidelines suggest not using these based on the SOX trial, which is the largest trial performed to date.[21,32] The SOX trial randomized 806 patients with first symptomatic proximal DVT to 30 to 40 mm Hg graduated elastic compression stocking or placebo stockings with less than 5 mm Hg compression. Primary outcome was development of postthrombotic syndrome at 2 years. There was no difference between active and placebo stocking groups using the specific Ginsberg scale (14.2% vs 12.7%) or the sensitive Villalta scale (52.6% vs 52.3%). A subsequent meta-analysis of 5 randomized trials, with the SOX trial representing more than half the patients, shows a 38% relative reduction in postthrombotic syndrome, although there was large statistical heterogeneity ($I^2 = 80\%$).[33]

VENOUS THROMBOEMBOLISM TREATMENT
Initial Anticoagulation

Initial anticoagulation (or acute anticoagulation) refers to anticoagulation choice at time of diagnosis. ACCP guidelines suggest DOACs over warfarin, and studies have demonstrated that DOACs have equal efficacy and improved safety.[21] The dosing of these various agents is reviewed in **Table 2**.

Vitamin K Antagonists

The first trial in 1960 that compared anticoagulant therapy with no anticoagulant therapy in patients with symptomatic DVT or PE suggested that 1.5 days of heparin and 14 days of vitamin K antagonist (VKA) therapy markedly reduced recurrent PE and mortality in patients with acute PE.[41] A 1992 randomized trial compared continuous intravenous heparin plus VKA versus VKA alone and was terminated early due to excess of symptomatic events in the VKA alone group.[42] Therefore, parenteral anticoagulation must be continued for at least 5 days and an International Normalized Ratio (INR) above 2 for 2 consecutive days.[43] However, ACCP does comment that if the INR exceeds the therapeutic range prematurely, it is acceptable to stop parenteral therapy before the patient has received 5 days of treatment.[44,45]

Table 2
Anticoagulation dosing for venous thromboembolsim

Anticoagulant	Initial Dose and Length	Maintenance Dose
Unfractionated Heparin[34]	• Weight Based: 80 units/kg bolus, then 18 units/kg/h (preferred)	Adjust infusion rate to maintain target laboratory values based on institutional protocol to maintain therapeutic aPTT 1.5–2.5 times the control
Low-Molecular-Weight Heparin (Enoxaparin)[35]	• 1 mg/kg twice daily (preferred) • 1.5 mg/kg QD can be used in nonobese patients • CrCl <30 mL/min: reduce to 1 mg/kg once daily	Same
Fondaparinux[36]	• 5 mg QD (<50 kg) • 7.5 mg QD (50–100 kg) • 10 mg QD (>100 kg)	Same
Apixaban[37]	• 10 mg BID first 7 d • CrCl ≤30 mL/min: has not been studied	5 mg BID
Dabigatran[38]	• 150 mg twice daily (after initial 5–10 d of parenteral anticoagulation) • CrCl ≤30 mL/min: has not been studied	Same
Rivaroxaban[39]	• 15 mg BID for the first 3 wk • CrCl <30 mL/min: avoid use	20 mg QD
Edoxaban[40]	• 60 mg once daily >60 kg • 30 mg once daily <60 kg or CrCl 15–50 mL/min (after initial 5–10 d of parenteral anticoagulation)	Same

Abbreviation: aPTT, activated partial thromboplastin time; CrCl, creatinine clearance.

Heparin, Low-Molecular-Weight Heparin, or Fondaparinux

ACCP guidelines suggest LMWH or fondaparinux over intravenous or subcutaneous unfractionated heparin (UFH).[44] A 2017 Cochrane meta-analysis of 29 randomized controlled trials comparing twice daily LMWH with UFH in patients with acute VTE demonstrated recurrence in 3.6% with LMWH versus 5.3% with UFH (OR 0.72 $P = .001$) and major bleeding rates of 1.1% LMWH versus 1.9% UFH (OR 0.58 $P = .02$).[46,47]

There are subsets of patients in whom IV UFH should still be the initial anticoagulant. Patients with renal failure creatinine clearance (CrCl) less than 30 mL/min have relative contraindications to LMWH, fondaparinux, and DOACs. Also, those who are hemodynamically unstable from massive PE and those who may need urgent discontinuation of anticoagulation should also be treated with IV UFH.[4] A weight-based dosing nomogram protocol is recommended over a non–weight-based protocol for IV UFH. A higher percentage of patients randomized to weight-adjusted dosing achieve a therapeutic activated partial thromboplastin time (aPTT) within 24 hours (97% vs 77%) without an increase in major bleeding.[34] The efficacy of IV UFH depends on achieving a critical therapeutic level within 24 hours of initiation, which is target aPTT ratio of 1.5 to 2.5 times control. A pooled analysis of 3 randomized trials showed an increased risk of recurrent VTE when a therapeutic aPTT was not achieved within 24 hours (23% vs 4%, $P = .02$).[48] Fondaparinux has been found to be comparable to LMWH for acute VTE treatment in the MATISSE trial with no difference in recurrent VTE, major bleeding, or mortality.[49] It also has the benefit of being able to be used in patients with history of heparin-induced thrombocytopenia.

Direct Oral Anticoagulants

The ACCP antithrombotic guidelines give a grade 2B suggestion for a DOAC over VKA therapy.[21] This suggestion is based on less bleeding with DOACs and greater convenience for patients and health care providers. The DOAC trials are summarized in **Table 3**.

To mitigate the high recurrence rate in the first several weeks of treatment, 2 different approaches were taken by trial investigators. Dabigatran and edoxaban were studied with at least 5 days of lead in (not overlap) with parenteral anticoagulation before DOAC initiation to help mitigate the high recurrence rate in the first week or so of therapy. Dabigatran and edoxaban require at least 5 days of parenteral anticoagulation with unfractionated heparin, LMWH, or fondaparinux and then parenteral anticoagulation is stopped and they are started.[50,51,55] Rivaroxaban was studied with a 50% increase of the daily dose for 3 weeks, whereas the apixaban trial used a 2-fold increase for 1 week.[52–54]

Long-Term Anticoagulation

Long-term anticoagulation refers to treatment during the initial 3 months. At 3 months the decision is made on whether to extend anticoagulation based on risk of recurrence and bleeding (**Table 4**).

A 2014 review of 6 trials including 27,023 patients with VTE compared DOACs with VKAs; recurrent VTE occurred in 2.0% of DOAC recipients versus 2.2% in VKA recipients. Treatment with a DOAC significantly reduced the risk of major bleeding (risk ratio 0.61 $P = .002$) as well as intracranial bleeding, fatal bleeding, and clinically relevant nonmajor bleeding.[56]

Extended Anticoagulation

Extended anticoagulation refers to treating indefinitely past 3-month standard long-term treatment. This decision must weigh the risk of VTE recurrence versus bleeding. Several

Table 3
Direct oral anticoagulant trials

Anticoagulant	Trial	Year	Recurrent VTE, DOAC vs Control	Safety Outcomes
Dabigatran	RE-COVER[50]	2009	Noninferiority 2.4% vs 2.1%	No significant difference in major bleeding Significant reduction in any bleeding in dabigatran (16.1% vs 21.9%)
Dabigatran	RE-COVER II[51]	2014	Noninferiority 2.3% vs 2.2%	No significant difference in major bleeding Significantly less any bleeding in dabigatran (15.6% vs 22.1%)
Rivaroxaban	EINSTEIN-DVT[52]	2010	Noninferiority 2.1% vs 3.0%	No significant difference in first major or clinically relevant nonmajor bleeding
Rivaroxaban	EINSTEIN-PE[53]	2012	Noninferiority 2.1% vs 1.8%	No significant difference in first major/clinically relevant nonmajor bleeding Significant decrease in major bleeding (1.1% vs 2.2%)
Apixaban	AMPLIFY[54]	2013	Noninferiority 2.3% vs 2.7%	Significantly less major bleeding (0.6% vs1.8%) Significantly less clinically relevant bleeding (3.8% vs 8.0%)
Edoxaban	Hokusai-VTE[55]	2013	Noninferiority 3.2% vs 3.5%	No significant difference in major bleeding Significantly less clinically relevant bleeding (8.5% vs10.3%)

scoring systems have been developed to assist in estimating VTE recurrence. The Men and HERDOO2 rule (hyperpigmentation, edema, or redness in either leg; D-dimer level ≥250 μg/L; obesity with body mass index ≥30; or Older age ≥65 years) estimated that women with an unprovoked VTE who have 0 of the criteria are low risk for recurrent VTE

Table 4
American College of Chest Physicians guideline anticoagulation length for proximal deep vein thrombosis or pulmonary embolism

Type of VTE	Bleeding Risk	Suggested Length	Grade of Evidence
Provoked by surgery	All	3 mo	1B
Provoked by a nonsurgical transient risk factor	Low/Moderate	3 mo	2B
	High	3 mo	1B
Unprovoked first VTE	Low	Extended (no stop date)	2B
Unprovoked first VTE	High	3 mo	1B
Unprovoked second VTE	Low	Extended (no stop date)	1B
Unprovoked second VTE	Moderate	Extended (no stop date)	2B
Unprovoked second VTE	High	3 mo	2B
Active cancer	Low/Moderate	Extended (no stop date)	1B
Active cancer	High	3 mo	2B

Data from Kearon C, Akl EA, Ornelas J, et al. Antithrombotic Therapy for VTE Disease: CHEST Guideline and Expert Panel Report. Chest 2016;149(2):315-352.

and stopping anticoagulation can be considered.[57] The DASH score uses risk factors of D-dimer, age, sex, and hormonal therapy for patient with an unprovoked VTE. A score less than or equal to 1 has a low annualized recurrence risk of 3.1%; anticoagulation may be able to be discontinued in these patients.[58] ACCP guidelines use 5 risk factors (**Table 5**) to guide the decision for extended anticoagulation.

Unlike atrial fibrillation in which the HAS-BLED score has been extensively validated, there are few robust bleeding risk assessment models for VTE. The RIETE score, which uses age greater than 75 years, recent bleeding, cancer, creatinine levels greater than 1.2 mg/dL, anemia, or pulmonary embolism, may be used to estimate bleeding risk.[59] The ACCP guidelines use bleeding risk factors (**Table 6**) to guide their recommendations for extended anticoagulation.

There have been multiple trials to evaluate extended anticoagulation, including anticoagulants versus placebo, anticoagulants versus aspirin, and aspirin versus placebo. Extended treatment with lower dose warfarin (INR 1.5–2.0), aspirin, or prophylactic dose DOAC have also been studied to mitigate bleeding, and selected trials are summarized (**Table 7**).

Usual dose warfarin (INR 2–3) is more effective and as safe as lower dose; prophylactic dose apixaban has less recurrence and no significant increase in major bleeding compared with placebo, and prophylactic dose rivaroxaban is more efficacious and as safe as aspirin. The use of lower prophylactic dose DOACs with their respective lower bleeding risk questions the traditional recurrent VTE threshold and therefore we recommend considering extended treatment of most patients.

SPECIAL POPULATIONS
Malignancy

Active malignancy represents a significant risk factor for VTE; the risk of proximal DVT or PE is 4- to 7-fold higher in patients with cancer compared with those without.[68] Initiation of anticoagulation further represents a challenge in this patient population, as they are significantly more likely to experience bleeding complications as well as VTE recurrence compared with the general population. Although guidelines have previously emphasized LMWH as first-line treatment, there is increasing evidence and acceptance for use of DOACs in the treatment of cancer-associated VTE. The Hokusai VTE Cancer study found edoxaban had similar net clinical benefit of recurrence and major bleeding as dalteparin with numerically less recurrence and more major bleeding with edoxaban.[69] Similarly, in the SELECT-D trial, rivaroxaban had a similar numeric trend of less recurrence and more bleeding with rivaroxaban compared with

Table 5
American College of Chest Physicians' estimated venous thromboembolism recurrence risk

Risk Factor	Recurrence Risk
Surgery	3% at 5 y
Transient nonsurgical (estrogen therapy, pregnancy, leg injury, flight of >8 h)	15% at 5 y
Unprovoked	30% at 5 y
Cancer	15% annual (not calculated at 5 y due to higher mortality)
Second unprovoked VTE	45% at 5 y

Data from Kearon C, Akl EA, Ornelas J, et al. Antithrombotic Therapy for VTE Disease: CHEST Guideline and Expert Panel Report. Chest 2016;149(2):315-352.

Table 6
American College of Chest Physicians' bleeding risk categories

Age >65 y	Diabetes
Age >75 y	Anemia
Previous bleeding	Antiplatelet therapy
Cancer	Poor anticoagulant control
Metastatic cancer	Comorbidity and reduced functional capacity
Renal failure	Recent surgery
Liver failure	Frequent falls
Thrombocytopenia	Alcohol abuse
Previous stroke	Nonsteroidal antiinflammatory drug
Risk Factors	
Low: 0 risk factors; Moderate: 1 risk factor; High: ≥2 risk factors	

Adapted from Kearon C, Akl EA, Ornelas J, et al. Antithrombotic Therapy for VTE Disease: CHEST Guideline and Expert Panel Report. Chest 2016;149(2):329; with permission.

dalteparin.[70] Both studies reported increased bleeding, mainly in patients with intact luminal gastrointestinal malignancies. More recently, the ADAM VTE trial studied the use of apixaban compared with dalteparin in patients with cancer and found lower rates of recurrent VTE with no increase in bleeding complications.[71] Given these findings, and in view of ISTH and NCCN guidelines, we recommend consideration of either of these agents for the treatment of cancer-related VTE, with very careful consideration of bleeding risk in those with gastroesophageal malignancy.[72–74]

Obesity

The use of DOACs in morbid obese patients (defined as a body mass index [BMI] >40 kg/m^2) remains controversial due to a paucity of clinical data in this population. To date, there has been no randomized clinical trial comparing vitamin K antagonist and DOACs dedicated to patients with BMI greater than 40 kg/m^2 for the treatment of acute VTE. Pharmacokinetic studies have indicated the challenge in using DOACs due to higher volume of distribution and lower mean peak concentration in patients weighing greater than 120 kg. Because of these obstacles, clinical guidance favors VKA over DOACs for patients with a BMI greater than 40 kg/m^2 or 120 kg or greater than 35 kg/m^2 or 120 kg.[75,76] In contrast, there have been retrospective studies investigating clinical outcomes with use of rivaroxaban, which found no increase in recurrent VTE or bleeding.[77] Further, the Dresden NOAC registry found elevated BMI is associated with a decrease in adverse events with use of DOACs, the so-called obesity paradox.[78]

Given the lack of data to support definitive recommendations in patient with acute VTE and BMI greater than 35 to 40 kg/m^2, it is suggested to use vitamin K antagonists in this population. In the appropriate clinical scenario, DOACs can be considered and management guided by DOAC levels according to ISTH guidance—anti-FXa levels for edoxaban, rivaroxaban, or apixaban or dilute thrombin time for dabigatran, although they are not readily available. Mass spectrometry drug levels can alternatively be used for all DOACs.[75]

Renal Failure

Chronic kidney disease represents an independent risk factor not only for VTE occurrence but also for bleeding complications during treatment. Patients with CrCl less

Table 7
Extended anticoagulation trials

Trial	Year	Anticoagulation	Control	Recurrent VTE Efficacy	Safety Outcomes
Kearon Seminal Study[60]	1999	Warfarin (additional 24 mo)	Placebo	Significantly reduced, 1.3% vs 27.4% per 100 person-years	No significant difference in major bleeding
PREVENT[61]	2003	Low-intensity Warfarin (INR 1.5–1.9)	Placebo	Significantly reduced, 2.6 vs 7.2 per 100 person-years	No significant difference in major bleeding
ELATE[62]	2003	Low-intensity Warfarin (INR 1.5–1.9)	Standard Warfarin (INR 2–3)	Significantly increased, 1.9 vs 0.7 per 100 person-years	No significant difference in any or major bleeding
EINSTEIN CHOICE[63]	2017	Rivaroxaban 20 mg	Aspirin	Significantly reduced, 1.5% vs 4.4%	No significant difference clinically relevant or major bleeding
	2017	Rivaroxaban 10 mg	Aspirin	Significantly reduced, 1.2% vs 4.4%	No significant difference in clinically relevant or major bleeding
AMPLIFY-EXT[64]	2013	Apixaban 2.5 mg	Placebo	Significantly reduced, 1.7% vs 8.8	No significant difference in major bleeding or clinically relevant nonmajor bleeding
	2013	Apixaban 5 mg	Placebo	Significantly reduced, 1.7% vs 8.8	No significant difference in major bleeding
RE-MEDY[65]	2013	Dabigatran	Warfarin	Noninferiority, 1.8% vs 1.3%	Increased clinically relevant nonmajor bleeding (1.82 RR)
RE-SONATE[65]	2013	Dabigatran	Placebo	Significantly reduced, 0.4% vs 5.6%	No significant difference in major bleeding Significant decreased major or clinically relevant bleeding, 5.6% vs10.2%
ASPIRE[66]	2012	Aspirin	Placebo	No significant difference	Significantly increased major or clinically relevant bleeding, 5.3% vs1.8%
WARFASA[67]	2012	Aspirin	Placebo	Significantly reduced, 6.6% vs 11.2%	No significant difference in major or clinically relevant nonmajor bleeding

than 30 mL/min, calculated with the Cockroff-Gualt equation using actual body weight, were excluded from trials that studied DOACs in the treatment of acute VTE.[79] Given the lack of data in this patient population, vitamin K antagonists are likely preferred for the treatment of VTE in patients with a CrCl less than 30 mL/min.

DISCLOSURE

S. Nair, N. Garza, M. George: nothing to declare. S. Kaatz: research support to institution. Consulting: Janssen, Pfizer, Portola, Roche, and Bristol Myers Squibb.

REFERENCES

1. Beckman MG, Hooper WC, Critchley SE, et al. Venous thromboembolism: a public health concern. Am J Prev Med 2010;38(4 Suppl):S495–501.
2. Mehta KD, Siddappa Malleshappa SK, Patel S, et al. Trends of inpatient venous thromboembolism in United States before and after the surgeon general's call to action. Am J Cardiol 2019;124(6):960–5.
3. Amin A, Deitelzweig S, Bucior I, et al. Frequency of hospital readmissions for venous thromboembolism and associated hospital costs and length of stay among acute medically ill patients in the US. J Med Econ 2019;22(11):1119–25.
4. Konstantinides SV, Meyer G, Becattini C, et al. 2019 ESC guidelines for the diagnosis and management of acute pulmonary embolism developed in collaboration with the European Respiratory Society (ERS). Eur Heart J 2020;41(4):543–603.
5. Aujesky D, Obrosky DS, Stone RA, et al. Derivation and validation of a prognostic model for pulmonary embolism. Am J Respir Crit Care Med 2005;172(8):1041–6.
6. Jimenez D, Aujesky D, Moores L, et al. Simplification of the pulmonary embolism severity index for prognostication in patients with acute symptomatic pulmonary embolism. Arch Intern Med 2010;170(15):1383–9.
7. Barco S, Mahmoudpour SH, Planquette B, et al. Prognostic value of right ventricular dysfunction or elevated cardiac biomarkers in patients with low-risk pulmonary embolism: a systematic review and meta-analysis. Eur Heart J 2019; 40(11):902–10.
8. Harjola VP, Mebazaa A, Celutkiene J, et al. Contemporary management of acute right ventricular failure: a statement from the Heart Failure Association and the Working Group on Pulmonary Circulation and Right Ventricular Function of the European Society of Cardiology. Eur J Heart Fail 2016;18(3):226–41.
9. Konstam MA, Kiernan MS, Bernstein D, et al. Evaluation and management of right-sided heart failure: a scientific statement from the American Heart Association. Circulation 2018;137(20):e578–622.
10. Yusuff HO, Zochios V, Vuylsteke A. Extracorporeal membrane oxygenation in acute massive pulmonary embolism: a systematic review. Perfusion 2015;30(8): 611–6.
11. Hao Q, Dong BR, Yue J, et al. Thrombolytic therapy for pulmonary embolism. CochraneDatabase Syst Rev 2018;(12):CD004437.
12. Lee T, Itagaki S, Chiang YP, et al. Survival and recurrence after acute pulmonary embolism treated with pulmonary embolectomy or thrombolysis in New York State, 1999 to 2013. J Thorac Cardiovasc Surg 2018;155(3):1084–90.e2.
13. Kuo WT, Banerjee A, Kim PS, et al. Pulmonary embolism response to fragmentation, embolectomy, and catheter thrombolysis (PERFECT): initial results from a prospective multicenter registry. Chest 2015;148(3):667–73.

14. Kucher N, Boekstegers P, Muller OJ, et al. Randomized, controlled trial of ultrasound-assisted catheter-directed thrombolysis for acute intermediate-risk pulmonary embolism. Circulation 2014;129(4):479–86.
15. Piazza G, Hohlfelder B, Jaff MR, et al. A prospective, single-arm, multicenter trial of ultrasound-facilitated, catheter-directed, low-dose fibrinolysis for acute massive and submassive pulmonary embolism: the SEATTLE II study. JACC Cardiovasc Interv 2015;8(10):1382–92.
16. Tu T, Toma C, Tapson VF, et al. A prospective, single-arm, multicenter trial of catheter-directed mechanical thrombectomy for intermediate-risk acute pulmonary embolism: the FLARE study. JACC Cardiovasc Interv 2019;12(9):859–69.
17. Sista A. Evaluating the Safety and Efficacy of the Indigo® Aspiration System in Acute Pulmonary Embolism. 2019. Available at: https://clinicaltrials.gov/ct2/show/NCT03218566. Accessed November 28, 2019.
18. Meyer G, Vicaut E, Danays T, et al. Fibrinolysis for patients with intermediate-risk pulmonary embolism. N Engl J Med 2014;370(15):1402–11.
19. Chatterjee S, Chakraborty A, Weinberg I, et al. Thrombolysis for pulmonary embolism and risk of all-cause mortality, major bleeding, and intracranial hemorrhage: a meta-analysis. JAMA 2014;311(23):2414–21.
20. Marti C, John G, Konstantinides S, et al. Systemic thrombolytic therapy for acute pulmonary embolism: a systematic review and meta-analysis. Eur Heart J 2015;36(10):605–14.
21. Kearon C, Akl EA, Ornelas J, et al. Antithrombotic therapy for VTE disease: CHEST guideline and expert panel report. Chest 2016;149(2):315–52.
22. Sharifi M, Bay C, Skrocki L, et al. Moderate pulmonary embolism treated with thrombolysis (from the "MOPETT" Trial). Am J Cardiol 2013;111(2):273–7.
23. Kiser TH, Burnham EL, Clark B, et al. Half-dose versus full-dose alteplase for treatment of pulmonary embolism. Crit Care Med 2018;46(10):1617–25.
24. Aujesky D, Roy PM, Verschuren F, et al. Outpatient versus inpatient treatment for patients with acute pulmonary embolism: an international, open-label, randomised, non-inferiority trial. Lancet 2011;378(9785):41–8.
25. Zondag W, Mos IC, Creemers-Schild D, et al. Outpatient treatment in patients with acute pulmonary embolism: the Hestia Study. J Thromb Haemost 2011;9(8):1500–7.
26. Bariteau A, Stewart LK, Emmett TW, et al. Systematic review and meta-analysis of outcomes of patients with subsegmental pulmonary embolism with and without anticoagulation treatment. Acad Emerg Med 2018;25(7):828–35.
27. Carrier M. A study to evaluate the safety of withholding anticoagulation in patients with subsegmental pe who have a negative serial bilateral lower extremity ultrasound (SSPE). 2011. Available at: https://clinicaltrials.gov/ct2/show/NCT01455818. Accessed November 27, 2019.
28. Kirkilesis G, KS, Bicknell C, et al. Treatment of distal deep vein thrombosis. 2019. Available at: https://www.cochrane.org/CD013422/PVD_treatment-distal-deep-vein-thrombosis. Accessed November 17, 2019.
29. Righini M, Galanaud JP, Guenneguez H, et al. Anticoagulant therapy for symptomatic calf deep vein thrombosis (CACTUS): a randomised, double-blind, placebo-controlled trial. Lancet Haematol 2016;3(12):e556–62.
30. Watson L, Broderick C, Armon MP. Thrombolysis for acute deep vein thrombosis. CochraneDatabase Syst Rev 2016;(11):CD002783.
31. Vedantham S, Goldhaber SZ, Julian JA, et al. Pharmacomechanical catheter-directed thrombolysis for deep-vein thrombosis. N Engl J Med 2017;377(23):2240–52.

32. Kahn SR, Shapiro S, Wells PS, et al. Compression stockings to prevent post-thrombotic syndrome: a randomised placebo-controlled trial. Lancet 2014; 383(9920):880–8.

33. Appelen D, van Loo E, Prins MH, et al. Compression therapy for prevention of post-thrombotic syndrome. CochraneDatabase Syst Rev 2017;(9):CD004174.

34. Raschke RA, Reilly BM, Guidry JR, et al. The weight-based heparin dosing nomogram compared with a "standard care" nomogram. A randomized controlled trial. Ann Intern Med 1993;119(9):874–81.

35. Lovenox® (enoxaparin sodium) [package insert] Paris, France : Sanofi-aventis; 2018.

36. ARIXTRA®(fondaparinux sodium) [package inset]. Brentford, UK: GlaxoSmithKline LLC; 2013.

37. ELIQUIS® (apixaban) [package insert]. New York, NY: Bristol-Myers Squibb Company; 2019.

38. PRADAXA® (dabigatran etexilate mesylate) [package insert]. Ingelheim am Rhein, Germany: Boehringer Ingelheim Pharmaceuticals; 2018.

39. XARELTO (rivaroxaban) [package insert]. Beerse, Belgium: Janssen Ortho; 2019.

40. SAVAYSA (edoxaban) [package insert].Tokyo, Japan: Daiichi Sankyo; 2019.

41. Barritt DW, Jordan SC. Anticoagulant drugs in the treatment of pulmonary embolism. A controlled trial. Lancet 1960;1(7138):1309–12.

42. Brandjes DP, Heijboer H, Buller HR, et al. Acenocoumarol and heparin compared with acenocoumarol alone in the initial treatment of proximal-vein thrombosis. N Engl J Med 1992;327(21):1485–9.

43. Leroyer C, Bressollette L, Oger E, et al. Early versus delayed introduction of oral vitamin K antagonists in combination with low-molecular-weight heparin in the treatment of deep vein thrombosis. a randomized clinical trial. The ANTENOX Study Group. Haemostasis 1998;28(2):70–7.

44. Kearon C, Akl EA, Comerota AJ, et al. Antithrombotic therapy for VTE disease: antithrombotic therapy and prevention of thrombosis, 9th ed: American College of Chest Physicians Evidence-Based Clinical Practice Guidelines. Chest 2012; 141(2 Suppl):e419S–96S.

45. Garcia DA, Baglin TP, Weitz JI, et al. Parenteral anticoagulants: antithrombotic therapy and prevention of thrombosis, 9th ed: American College of Chest Physicians evidence-based clinical practice guidelines. Chest 2012;141(2 Suppl): e24S–43S.

46. Robertson L, Jones LE. Fixed dose subcutaneous low molecular weight heparins versus adjusted dose unfractionated heparin for the initial treatment of venous thromboembolism. CochraneDatabase Syst Rev 2017;(2):CD001100.

47. van Dongen CJ, MacGillavry MR, Prins MH. Once versus twice daily LMWH for the initial treatment of venous thromboembolism. CochraneDatabase Syst Rev 2005;(3):CD003074.

48. Hull RD, Raskob GE, Brant RF, et al. Relation between the time to achieve the lower limit of the APTT therapeutic range and recurrent venous thromboembolism during heparin treatment for deep vein thrombosis. Arch Intern Med 1997; 157(22):2562–8.

49. Buller HR, Davidson BL, Decousus H, et al. Fondaparinux or enoxaparin for the initial treatment of symptomatic deep venous thrombosis: a randomized trial. Ann Intern Med 2004;140(11):867–73.

50. Schulman S, Kearon C, Kakkar AK, et al. Dabigatran versus warfarin in the treatment of acute venous thromboembolism. N Engl J Med 2009;361(24):2342–52.

51. Schulman S, Kakkar AK, Goldhaber SZ, et al. Treatment of acute venous throm-boembolism with dabigatran or warfarin and pooled analysis. Circulation 2014; 129(7):764–72.

52. Bauersachs R, Berkowitz SD, Brenner B, et al. Oral rivaroxaban for symptomatic venous thromboembolism. N Engl J Med 2010;363(26):2499–510.

53. Buller HR, Prins MH, Lensin AW, et al. Oral rivaroxaban for the treatment of symp-tomatic pulmonary embolism. N Engl J Med 2012;366(14):1287–97.

54. Agnelli G, Buller HR, Cohen A, et al. Oral apixaban for the treatment of acute venous thromboembolism. N Engl J Med 2013;369(9):799–808.

55. Hokusai VTEI, Buller HR, Decousus H, et al. Edoxaban versus warfarin for the treatment of symptomatic venous thromboembolism. N Engl J Med 2013; 369(15):1406–15.

56. van Es N, Coppens M, Schulman S, et al. Direct oral anticoagulants compared with vitamin K antagonists for acute venous thromboembolism: evidence from phase 3 trials. Blood 2014;124(12):1968–75.

57. Rodger MA, Le Gal G, Anderson DR, et al. Validating the HERDOO2 rule to guide treatment duration for women with unprovoked venous thrombosis: multinational prospective cohort management study. BMJ 2017;356:j1065.

58. Tosetto A, Iorio A, Marcucci M, et al. Predicting disease recurrence in patients with previous unprovoked venous thromboembolism: a proposed prediction score (DASH). J Thromb Haemost 2012;10(6):1019–25.

59. Ruiz-Gimenez N, Suarez C, Gonzalez R, et al. Predictive variables for major bleeding events in patients presenting with documented acute venous thrombo-embolism. Findings from the RIETE Registry. Thromb Haemost 2008;100(1):26–31.

60. Kearon C, Gent M, Hirsh J, et al. A comparison of three months of anticoagulation with extended anticoagulation for a first episode of idiopathic venous thrombo-embolism. N Engl J Med 1999;340(12):901–7.

61. Ridker PM, Goldhaber SZ, Danielson E, et al. Long-term, low-intensity warfarin therapy for the prevention of recurrent venous thromboembolism. N Engl J Med 2003;348(15):1425–34.

62. Kearon C, Ginsberg JS, Kovacs MJ, et al. Comparison of low-intensity warfarin therapy with conventional-intensity warfarin therapy for long-term prevention of recurrent venous thromboembolism. N Engl J Med 2003;349(7):631–9.

63. Weitz JI, Lensing AWA, Prins MH, et al. Rivaroxaban or aspirin for extended treat-ment of venous thromboembolism. N Engl J Med 2017;376(13):1211–22.

64. Agnelli G, Buller HR, Cohen A, et al. Apixaban for extended treatment of venous thromboembolism. N Engl J Med 2013;368(8):699–708.

65. Schulman S, Kearon C, Kakkar AK, et al. Extended use of dabigatran, warfarin, or placebo in venous thromboembolism. N Engl J Med 2013;368(8):709–18.

66. Brighton TA, Eikelboom JW, Mann K, et al. Low-dose aspirin for preventing recur-rent venous thromboembolism. N Engl J Med 2012;367(21):1979–87.

67. Becattini C, Agnelli G, Schenone A, et al. Aspirin for preventing the recurrence of venous thromboembolism. N Engl J Med 2012;366(21):1959–67.

68. Schmaier AA, Ambesh P, Campia U. Venous thromboembolism and cancer. Curr Cardiol Rep 2018;20(10):89.

69. Raskob GE, van Es N, Verhamme P, et al. Edoxaban for the Treatment of cancer-associated venous thromboembolism. N Engl J Med 2018;378(7):615–24.

70. Young AM, Marshall A, Thirlwall J, et al. Comparison of an oral factor Xa inhibitor with low molecular weight heparin in patients with cancer with venous thrombo-embolism: results of a randomized trial (SELECT-D). J Clin Oncol 2018;36(20): 2017–23.

71. McBane R 2nd, Wysokinski WE, Le-Rademacher JG, et al. Apixaban and dalteparin in active malignancy-associated venous thromboembolism: the ADAM VTE trial. J Thromb Haemost 2020;18(2):411–21.

72. Streiff MB, Holmstrom B, Angelini D, et al. NCCN guidelines insights: cancer-associated venous thromboembolic disease, version 2.2018. J Natl Compr Canc Netw 2018;16(11):1289.

73. Khorana AA, Noble S, Lee AYY, et al. Role of direct oral anticoagulants in the treatment of cancer-associated venous thromboembolism: guidance from the SSC of the ISTH. J Thromb Haemost 2018;16(9):1891–4.

74. Key NS, Khorana AA, Kuderer NM, et al. Venous thromboembolism prophylaxis and treatment in patients with cancer: ASCO clinical practice guideline update. J Clin Oncol 2020;38(5):496–520.

75. Martin K, Beyer-Westendorf J, Davidson BL, et al. Use of the direct oral anticoagulants in obese patients: guidance from the SSC of the ISTH. J Thromb Haemost 2016;14(6):1308–13.

76. Burnett AE, Mahan CE, Vazquez SR, et al. Guidance for the practical management of the direct oral anticoagulants (DOACs) in VTE treatment. J Thromb Thrombolysis 2016;41(1):206–32.

77. Di Nisio M, Vedovati MC, Riera-Mestre A, et al. Treatment of venous thromboembolism with rivaroxaban in relation to body weight. A sub-analysis of the EINSTEIN DVT/PE studies. Thromb Haemost 2016;116(4):739–46.

78. Tittl L, Endig S, Marten S, et al. Impact of BMI on clinical outcomes of NOAC therapy in daily care - Results of the prospective Dresden NOAC Registry (NCT01588119). Int J Cardiol 2018;262:85–91.

79. Giustozzi M, Franco L, Vedovati MC, et al. Safety of direct oral anticoagulants versus traditional anticoagulants in venous thromboembolism. J Thromb Thrombolysis 2019;48(3):439–53.

Acute Liver Injury and Decompensated Cirrhosis

James F. Crismale, MD*, Scott L. Friedman, MD

KEYWORDS

- Acute liver injury • Acute liver failure • Decompensated cirrhosis
- Hepatic encephalopathy • Variceal hemorrhage • Ascites • Hepatorenal syndrome

KEY POINTS

- In the hospitalized patient, acute liver injury often results from drug-induced liver injury or hypoxic, viral, or autoimmune hepatitis.
- Acute liver failure is a distinct clinical syndrome defined by the development of hepatic encephalopathy within 26 weeks of the onset of liver injury, and it has a high mortality without liver transplantation.
- Transition from compensated to decompensated cirrhosis is defined by the development of complications of portal hypertension that often necessitate hospitalization, including hepatic encephalopathy, variceal hemorrhage, and ascites.

ACUTE LIVER INJURY AND ACUTE LIVER FAILURE
Introduction

Acute liver injury (ALI) is defined by the development of abnormal liver chemistries – alanine aminotransferase (ALT), aspartate aminotransferase (AST), or alkaline phosphatase (ALP) – in a patient without prior liver disease, and in whom the liver abnormalities have been present for less than 6 months. True liver function tests including bilirubin, albumin, and prothrombin time/international normalized ratio (PT/INR) may become abnormal as ALI progresses and liver function becomes impaired. With further hepatocyte loss, impaired clearance of ammonia and other metabolites contribute to the development of hepatic encephalopathy (HE). The development of HE in a patient with ALI, coagulopathy, and jaundice marks the progression from ALI to acute liver failure (ALF), a rare condition with a high risk of death without liver transplantation (LT). The diagnosis of ALF requires:

- ALI with or without jaundice in a patient without prior liver disease
- International normalized ratio (INR) of at least 1.5
- Hepatic encephalopathy that develops within 26 weeks of disease onset

Division of Liver Diseases, Department of Medicine, Icahn School of Medicine at Mount Sinai, One Gustave L. Levy Place, Box 1109, New York, NY 10029, USA
* Corresponding author.
E-mail address: James.crismale@mountsinai.org

Med Clin N Am 104 (2020) 647–662
https://doi.org/10.1016/j.mcna.2020.02.010
0025-7125/20/© 2020 Elsevier Inc. All rights reserved.

Although most ALI cases will resolve before they progress to ALF, it is essential for the hospitalist to be aware of how these conditions are defined and what interventions may be available to improve outcomes for these patients.[1]

Initial Classification and Assessment of Etiology

In a patient presenting with ALI, it is essential to determine[1]: whether ALF is present, as triage and patient management change rapidly, and[2] to assess the etiology of the ALI, as this can inform management. Liver enzyme abnormalities can be classified as follows[2]:

- Hepatocellular: ALT at least 3 times the upper limit of normal (ULN), ALP less than 2 times the ULN
- Cholestatic: ALP greater than 2 times the ULN, ALT less than 3 times the ULN
- Mixed: ALT at least 3 times the ULN and ALP greater than 2 times the ULN

The pattern of liver enzyme abnormalities is helpful in determining a differential diagnosis and may have prognostic significance, with hepatocellular ALI more likely to present acutely and resolve within days to weeks, while cholestatic or mixed ALI may present in a more subacute fashion and resolve more slowly (**Table 1**).[2] The magnitude of liver enzyme elevation also provides important clues. Massive elevations (eg, ALT >10,000) are noted in only a few conditions: acetaminophen (APAP) or other drug toxicity, acute viral hepatitis, autoimmune hepatitis, ischemic/hypoxic hepatitis, or biliary disease with acute duct obstruction.

Following initial assessment and triage, a thorough history and physical examination are essential. Patients may be asymptomatic (with laboratory tests checked for unrelated reasons) or may initially present with vague symptoms, including fever, fatigue, malaise, right upper quadrant (RUQ) pain, jaundice, or nausea and vomiting. The history should focus on assessment of risk factors for various etiologies of liver disease (**Table 2**). The physical examination should include an assessment for RUQ tenderness, hepatosplenomegaly, jaundice, and adenopathy. Evidence of sarcopenia, ascites, spider angiomata, caput medusae, or other signs of portal hypertension may prompt a diagnostic workup for decompensated chronic liver disease rather than ALI.

Additional laboratory testing is often necessary to identify the etiology and to assess the severity of liver disease (see **Table 2**).[3] Severity of ALI can be determined by serial monitoring of bilirubin, INR, factor V, and fibrinogen. Liver-related blood tests should be checked serially. If the patient is jaundiced or coagulopathic, then more frequent monitoring (every 4–6 hours) is necessary to guide management and to monitor for the development of ALF.

All patients with ALI should receive liver imaging. An RUQ Doppler ultrasound is typically performed first. This is useful in assessment of the hepatic parenchyma, bile ducts, and patency of the portal and hepatic veins. If malignant hepatic infiltration is

Table 1
Classification of liver injury in acute liver injury

Hepatocellular	Cholestatic	Mixed
• Acetaminophen toxicity	• Drug-induced	• Drug-induced
• Drug-induced	• Infiltrative	• Alcohol-related
• Ischemic	• Congestive hepatopathy	• Multifactorial
• Viral	• Biliary obstruction	
• Autoimmune		
• Acute biliary obstruction		

Table 2
Important clinical and laboratory features of different causes of acute liver injury

Classification	Pertinent H&P Findings	Pertinent Laboratory Testing
Viral	<ul><li>History of viral hepatitis</li><li>Immunization history (hepatitis A and B)</li><li>HAV – recent travel to endemic/epidemic area, recent sick contacts, men who have sex with men (MSM)[3]</li><li>HBV – persons from endemic areas, recent travel to an endemic are, persons who inject drugs (PWID), MSM, persons receiving immunosuppressive or chemotherapy, patient with end-stage renal disease (ESRD), persons with HIV, >1 sex partner in the past 6 mo, health care worker, any possible exposure to blood/bodily fluids of another individual with known HBV[4]</li><li>HCV – MSM, PWID, >1 sex partner in the last 6 mo, ESRD, any possible exposure to blood/bodily fluids of another individual with known HCV[5]</li><li>HEV – recent travel to endemic area (eg, southeast Asia), recent contact with pigs, wild boar, or deer[6]</li><li>Nonhepatotropic viruses (eg, EBV, CMV, VZV, HSV) – recent/current immunosuppression</li></ul>	<ul><li>Hepatitis A virus (HAV) immunoglobulin M (IgM)</li><li>HBcAb IgM</li><li>HBsAg</li><li>Hepatitis B virus (HBV) DNA</li><li>HDV Ag/RNA (if + HBV testing)</li><li>Hepatitis C virus (HCV) RNA</li><li>HCV Ab</li><li>Hepatitis E virus (HEV) IgM</li><li>HEV IgG</li><li>HSV IgM</li><li>Varicella zoster visur (VZV) IgM</li><li>Epstein-Barr virus (EBV), cytomegalovirus (CMV), herpes simplex virus (HSV) PCR</li></ul>
Autoimmune	<ul><li>Personal or family history of autoimmune disease, eg, Hashimoto thyroiditis, celiac disease, type I diabetes mellitus</li></ul>	<ul><li>Antinuclear antibody</li><li>Quantitative immunoglobulin G (IgG)</li><li>Anti-smooth muscle Ab</li><li>Anti-liver kidney microsomal Ab</li><li>Anti-soluble liver antigen antibody</li><li>Anti-nuclear cytoplasmic antibody</li></ul>
Drug	<ul><li>Recent acetaminophen use, including details about dosage and frequency of use</li><li>Current or recent prescription medications, including time of initiation and discontinuation</li><li>Recent antibiotic use (even if short duration)</li><li>Current or recent over the counter and/or herbal and dietary supplement (HDS) use</li></ul>	<ul><li>APAP level</li><li>Urinary toxicology</li></ul>

(continued on next page)

Table 2 (continued)		
Classification	**Pertinent H&P Findings**	**Pertinent Laboratory Testing**
Gallstone	• Personal or family history of gallstone disease • History of inflammatory bowel disease • History of oral contraceptive use	• None
Other	• Personal/family history of clotting disorders (assessing for vascular causes of ALI including Budd-Chiari syndrome) • Family history of metabolic liver disease • Personal history of unexplained or recent-onset neuropsychiatric symptoms (eg, Wilson disease) • History of solid malignancy or lymphoma (risk of malignant hepatic infiltration)	• Ceruloplasmin • 24-h urine copper

suspected, then contrast-enhanced cross-sectional imaging should be performed, although it should be noted that in a multicenter series of patients presenting with malignant infiltration as the etiology of acute liver failure, only 44% had tumor identified on imaging. The diagnosis of Budd-Chiari syndrome also requires imaging confirmation. Although Doppler-based ultrasonography has a sensitivity of up to 75% in experienced hands in identifying hepatic vein occlusion, it is operator dependent; therefore, contrast-enhanced cross-sectional imaging may be preferred.[3] Liver biopsy remains the gold standard for diagnosis and may be pursued if noninvasive testing is unrevealing, or if the suspected diagnosis based on serologic and imaging tests does not accord with the clinical history.

Management by Etiology

Drug-induced liver injury

Drug-induced liver injury (DILI) is the most common etiology of liver enzyme elevation in hospitalized patients and is responsible for greater than 50% of cases of ALF. APAP is responsible for 46% of ALF cases overall.[4,5] It is therefore essential that any assessment of abnormal liver chemistries in the hospitalized patient begin with a thorough medication history, including those that have been started during hospitalization. The pattern of liver enzyme elevation can be used to categorize the type of injury and to narrow down the list of potential etiologic agents (**Table 3**).[2]

DILI may also be categorized as dose-dependent or idiosyncratic. The prototype of dose-dependent hepatotoxicity is APAP-induced DILI, which may be seen when daily ingestion exceeds 7.5 to 10 g/d. Lower doses may be sufficient to induce ALI among patients with additional risk factors, including starvation or chronic alcohol use, which lead to depletion of intrahepatic glutathione stores and leave hepatocytes susceptible to oxidative injury from APAP metabolites. Medications that induce cytochrome P450 such as cimetidine or phenobarbital can alter APAP metabolism and lead to accumulation of toxic intermediaries and ALI, even with standard doses of APAP. Progression to ALF occurs in up to 9.1% of patients following APAP overdose. Measurement of

Table 3
Drugs causing typical patterns of drug-induced liver injury

Hepatocellular	Cholestatic	Mixed
• APAP	• Anabolic steroids	• Phenytoin
• Isoniazid	• Oral contraceptives	• Lamotrigine
• Allopurinol	• Cephalosporins	• Nonsteroidal anti-inflammatory
• Disulfram	• Rifampin	drugs (NSAIDs)
• Ephedra	• Amoxicillin/clavulanic acid	
• Green tea extract		

serum APAP level should be performed, but as the half-life of APAP is approximately 5.4 hours, a negative APAP level does not rule out recent ingestion.[6]

APAP-induced ALI typically manifests with extreme elevation in ALT and AST (sometimes >10,000) within 72 hours from the time of initial ingestion. This elevation is often accompanied by evidence of elevated bilirubin and INR that occurs within 72 to 96 hours following ingestion. If left untreated, ALF may result. Prompt administration of intravenous N-acetyl cysteine (NAC) is associated with a greater than 75% transplant-free survival (TFS).[5]

In contrast to APAP toxicity, idiosyncratic DILI occurs independent of drug dose. The most common classes of drugs implicated are antimicrobials followed by HDS. The prototypical form of idiosyncratic DILI is seen with isoniazid, where 10% to 20% of patients taking the drug at a therapeutic dose may develop liver enzyme abnormalities. The mechanism of injury appears to be direct hepatotoxicity caused by accumulation of a toxic intermediary. In contrast, amoxicillin/ clavulanc acid-induced DILI is thought to have an immunoallergenic mechanism, with the clavulanate component responsible for the abnormal host response.[4] There may be a latency of onset of up to 8 weeks. In contrast to APAP overdose, there is no specific antidote for idiosyncratic DILI, and management is supportive following discontinuation of the culprit agent.

Viral hepatitis
HAV causes a self-limited hepatitis. It is transmitted via the fecal-oral route and has an incubation period of about 2 to 6 weeks. Symptoms are those of acute hepatitis, with nonspecific gastrointestinal (GI) complaints, RUQ pain or discomfort, jaundice, scleral icterus, pruritus, and dark urine. A positive anti-HAV IgM antibody is suggestive of acute infection, while a positive IgG appears as clinical infection resolves. The disease is self-limited and will resolve with supportive treatment. Although rare (<1% of cases), it can progress to ALF, so vigilance is necessary.[5]

HEV is also transmitted via the fecal-oral route. The diagnosis of acute HEV infection can be made via detection of HEV IgM and HEV RNA, although the latter is not widely available. While it was previously thought to only be found in developing countries (especially those in southeast Asia), its prevalence is increasing in high-income countries also (current seroprevalence in the United States is 8.1%). Only 5% of patients with acute HEV become symptomatic; among those who do, the clinical course of acute HEV is typically self-limited. However, acute HEV can be severe, necessitating close monitoring[7] HEV infection can become chronic in immunocompromised patients, and can be treated with a combination of ribavirin and a reduction in immunosuppression.

HBV is transmitted via parenteral or sexual contact and can cause an acute symptomatic hepatitis in adults. Diagnosis is made via identification of anti-HBc IgM along with HBsAg and HBV DNA. In adults it resolves spontaneously in greater than 95% of cases, without the development of chronic HBV or the need for antiviral therapy.[8,9] ALF occurs in less than 1% of patients. Antiviral therapy may be helpful in patients with ALF, although ALF rarely reverses with antiviral therapy alone. Agents indicated for the treatment of both acute and chronic HBV include the nucleotide analogues entecavir and tenofovir.

Immunocompromised patients are at risk for reactivation of HBV infection, especially if they have had prior HBV exposure and are HBcAb-positive (with or without HBsAb) or HBsAg-positive. Patients should therefore be tested for HBsAg, HBcAb, and HBsAb prior to initiation of any immunosuppressive therapy.

Autoimmune hepatitis
Up to 25% of patients diagnosed with autoimmune hepatitis (AIH) may present with a severe presentation of the disease. This may represent an acute flare of chronic AIH that was previously undiagnosed, or a true acute onset of AIH. In acute presentations of the disease, typical autoimmune markers such as antismooth muscle antibodies may be undetectable, so a high index of suspicion is necessary. Liver biopsy may be necessary to establish the diagnosis. Corticosteroids are the mainstay of treatment for AIH and should be initiated only after expert consultation with gastroenterology/hepatology, especially if synthetic dysfunction is present. Extended high-dose corticosteroid therapy in a patient with ALF may predispose an already susceptible patient to a greater risk of infection, both before and after transplantation. Mortality in severe acute AIH ranges from 19% to 45%.[10]

Ischemic/hypoxic hepatitis
Also known as shock liver, ischemic or hypoxic hepatitis occurs when the dual blood supply to the liver (via the portal vein and hepatic artery) is compromised in the setting of systemic hypotension and passive hepatic congestion. Despite the association with hypotension, a preceding hypotensive event is variably identified. A predisposing acute cardiac event is identified in 78.2% of patients. Mortality in this condition is high (50%) but is most often related to the underlying condition rather than ALF, where the rate of spontaneous recovery is 71%.[11]

Other etiologies
Interventions for ALI resulting from less common etiologies are listed in **Table 4**.

Acute Liver Failure

Diagnosis and classification
As noted previously, ALF is a distinct clinical entity wherein ALI leads to rapid synthetic dysfunction, coagulopathy (INR >1.5), and HE within 26 weeks of symptom onset. ALF is a rare condition, with fewer than 2000 cases in the United States per year. Because of its rarity, patients with ALF account for only approximately 1% to3% of patients on the LT waiting list. In the United States, ALF from APAP overdose is most common (49%) followed by non-APAP DILI (11.1%) and AIH (8.4%).

The onset of ALF is often followed by the development of multiorgan dysfunction, most problematic of which is cerebral failure, which results from the development of cerebral edema. Death may subsequently result from brainstem herniation or global hypoxic cerebral injury (**Fig. 1**). The natural history of ALF is a study in the balance between hepatic necrosis and regeneration. With modern supportive care, up to 50% of patients with ALF are able to survive without LT, while 23% undergo LT, and 30% succumb.

Table 4
Specific interventions for various etiologies of acute liver injury

Etiology	Etiology-Directed Therapy
Acetaminophen	N-Acetylcysteine
Viral hepatitis	
HBV	Tenofovir, entecavir
HEV	Ribavirin
HAV	–
HSV/VZV	Acyclovir
EBV	–
Dengue, yellow fever, and similar diseases	–
Metabolic liver disease	
Wilson disease	Plasmapheresis, CVVH
Acute fatty liver of pregnancy	Delivery of fetus
Autoimmune hepatitis	Corticosteroids
Vascular	
Ischemic hepatitis	Resuscitation
Heat stroke	Targeted temperature management
Budd-Chiari syndrome	Thrombolysis, stenting, TIPS
Amanita toxicity	Charcoal (if early), penicillin G, silibilin

The clinical course of ALF can be characterized by the time from symptom onset to the development of hepatic encephalopathy as hyperacute (within 7 days), acute (8–28 days), or subacute (5–12 weeks).[1] ALF caused by APAP overdose represents the prototypical presentation of hyperacute liver failure; while dramatic, patients presenting with hyperacute ALF may have the greatest chance for TFS, with spontaneous recovery occurring in up to 75%. Examples of acute ALF and subacute ALF include acute or reactivated HBV infection and idiosyncratic DILI, respectively. Patients who present with subacute ALF have a lower TFS, ranging from 24.1% to 33.3%.

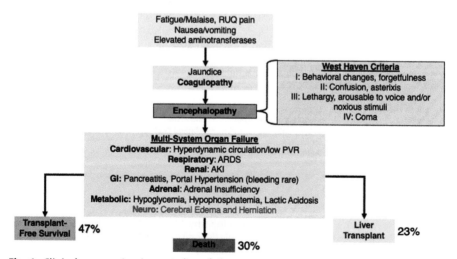

Fig. 1. Clinical progression in acute liver failure.

Initial management

All patients with ALF should be managed in the intensive care unit (ICU) setting and preferably transferred to a transplant center. Other initial steps in management include

- Infectious workup: blood and urine cultures, chest radiograph
- Neurologic monitoring every 1 to 2 hours
- Volume resuscitation with crystalloid
- Dextrose-containing solutions should be given to patients with hypoglycemia, which may result from poor oral intake and impaired gluconeogenesis
  - For those with suspected APAP-ALF: intravenous NAC; NB: intravenous NAC has been associated with improved TFS among patients with non-APAP ALF and grade I-II HE, and should be administered to these patients also[12]

Neurologic management

Neurologic failure related to brainstem herniation or global hypoxic injury is the most common cause of death among patients presenting with ALF. Clinically, HE in ALF is graded via the West Haven criteria (**Fig. 2**). Up to 75% of patients who develop grade IV HE develop intracranial hypertension (ICH), the clinical manifestation of cerebral edema. Higher ammonia levels at admission (>200 μmol/L) correlate with the development of ICH. Lactulose administration is considered ineffective in ALF, as NH_3 is generated too rapidly in ALF to be eliminated via the stool.[13]

General measures aimed at the reduction of ICH should be instituted for all patients once HE is detected:

- Early consultation with neurocritical care to assist with patient monitoring and management
- Place patients in a quiet room with minimal stimuli, including deep suctioning
- Head-of-bed should be elevated to 30°
- Sedation (short-acting agents including fentanyl or propofol) and intubation once grade III-IV HE develops

The gold standard for monitoring for the development of ICH is via placement of an intracranial pressure (ICP) monitor, although many LT programs avoid using invasive ICP monitoring because of the risk of intracranial hemorrhage. Further, ICP monitoring does not alter 21-day mortality. Noninvasive methods for ICP monitoring include

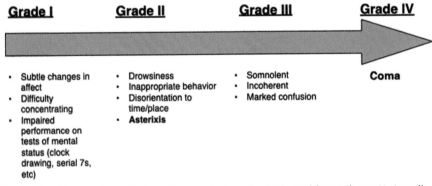

Fig. 2. West Haven criteria for hepatic encephalopathy. (*Adapted from* Vilstrup H, Amodio P, Bajaj J, et al. Hepatic encephalopathy in chronic liver disease: 2014 Practice guideline by the American Association for the Study of Liver Diseases and the European Association for the Study of the Liver. Hepatology 2014;60(2):719; with permission.)

measurement of optic nerve sheath diameter and estimation of ICP from transcranial Doppler.

If increased ICH develops, mannitol and hypertonic saline may both be used to draw water out of astrocytes and other glial cells and thereby reduce cerebral edema.[3] Hyperventilation to achieve a reduction in $Paco_2$ (target 25–30 mm Hg) may lead to cerebral vasoconstriction, possibly reducing vasogenic cerebral edema.[3]

Infection
Sepsis is the second most common cause of death among patients with ALF. Approximately 35% of patients with ALF develop bacteremia; the most common organisms are gram-negative (52%). Fungemia is a concern among patients with ALF, especially for patients on renal replacement therapy or those in the ICU for more than 7 days. Because patients in ALF may present with evidence of systemic inflammation, hypotension, and tachycardia, it may be difficult to distinguish when infection is present. Any deterioration in clinical status (eg, worsening encephalopathy or renal failure) should trigger a search for infection and the initiation of broad-spectrum antibiotics, with particular agents determined by local patterns of resistance and the hospital's antibiogram.[14]

Coagulopathy
Elevation in the INR is a key laboratory feature of ALF that results from deficient hepatic synthesis of vitamin K-dependent clotting factors. INR elevation alone does not accurately convey the risk of bleeding in ALF caused by coexistent deficits in anticlotting factors such as protein C and S, which lead to a rebalanced coagulation. Platelet count may serve as a better indicator of bleeding risk, with a platelet count of less than 60×10^3 per mm^3 associated with reduced thrombin generation and an increased bleeding risk. Prophylactic transfusion of products to correct coagulation parameters is not recommended, although it may be necessary prior to invasive procedures such as central line placement or placement of an ICP monitor.[15]

Renal failure
Acute kidney injury (AKI) occurs in up to 40% to 80% of patients with ALF, and develops because of a combination of volume depletion leading to prerenal azotemia and/or a hepatorenal-like syndrome resulting from vasodilatory shock, with or without underlying sepsis. AKI is associated with worse 21-day overall survival among patients with ALF, especially if renal replacement therapy (RRT) is required.

Transplantation
LT may be the only option for life-saving therapy for certain patients with ALF, although predicting which patients will require LT versus those who will survive with supportive care alone is challenging. Several scoring systems have been utilized to determine the risk of mortality and the need for LT in patients with ALF (**Table 5**). Hypophosphatemia portends high likelihood of spontaneous recovery in ALF, and is thought to be related to rapid uptake of inorganic phosphorous by the liver as a large amount of adenosine triphosphate is utilized in the regeneration process.[16]

Evaluation for LT is begun once the patient meets medical criteria for ALF, with a goal to complete the transplant evaluation and place the patient on the waiting list as rapidly as possible. The presence of uncontrolled sepsis or irreversible neurologic injury may contraindicate LT.[17] Post-LT outcomes for patients with ALF are generally good, with approximately 80% survival 1-year after LT.

Table 5
Scoring systems in acute liver failure

Score	Performance Characteristics	Comments
King's College Criteria – APAP • Arterial pH <7.3 or • 3 of the following: ○ HE grade >3 ○ INR >6.5 ○ Serum Cr >3.4 King's College Criteria – non-APAP • INR >6.5 or • 3 of 5 of the following: ○ Age <10 or >40 y ○ Jaundice to HE >7 d ○ Bilirubin >17 mg/dL ○ INR >3.5	For in-hospital mortality[16] • Sensitivity 59% (56%–62%) • Specificity 79% (77%–81%) • Positive likelihood ratio 2.5 (2.0–3.2) • Negative likelihood ratio 0.54 (0.46–0.64) • AUC 0.76	
MELD	For in-hospital mortality[16] • Sensitivity 74% (71%–77%) • Specificity 67% (64%–69%) • Positive likelihood ratio 2.4 (2.0–3.0) • Negative likelihood ratio 0.38 (0.31–0.46) AUC 0.78	Variable cutoffs across studies, ranging 25–37 NB: Original MELD, not MELD-Na
US ALF Study Group Model • Logit TFS = 2.67– 0.95(HE[a]) + 1.56(Etiology[a]) - 1.25(Vasopressor Use[a]) - 0.70 (ln bilirubin) - 1.35 (ln INR) • Predicted TFS = 1/(1 + e^(−1)*Logit TFS))	• C statistical = 0.84, 95% CI 0.82–0.87 • AUROC = 0.84 At threshold of 80% predicted TFS: • Sensitivity 37.1% (32.5%–41.8%) • Specificity 95.3% (92.9%–97.1%) • Positive predictive value 88.6% (83.1%–92.8%) • Negative predictive value 60.5% (63.1%–69.4%)	Encephalopathy Grade 1–2 = 0 Grade 3–4 = 1 Etiology Unfavorable = 0 Favorable = 1 Vasopressor use No = 0 Yes = 1

[a] Predicts 21-d transplant-free survival, not mortality.

PORTAL HYPERTENSION AND DECOMPENSATED LIVER DISEASE

In contrast to ALF, patients with end-stage liver disease (ESLD) related to cirrhosis are often hospitalized with complications of portal hypertension, including ascites, variceal hemorrhage, hepatic encephalopathy, and acute kidney injury caused by the hepatorenal syndrome.[18] The Child-Turcotte-Pugh (CTP) score and the Model for End-Stage Liver Disease (MELD) are used to predict mortality among patients with ESLD. The CTP score is currently used for assessing perioperative risk among patients with cirrhosis, while the MELD score is used for prioritizing patients on the LT waiting list given its ability to predict short-term (ie, 90-day) mortality (**Table 6**).[19] In 2016 the predictive value of the MELD score was augmented by the addition of serum sodium (SNa) as a covariable (**Table 7**).[20] LT provides a survival benefit among decompensated cirrhotic patients once MELD reaches 15.

Table 6 Child-Turcotte-Pugh score	Points		
	1	**2**	**3**
Encephalopathy	None	Grade 1–2	Grade 3–4
Ascites	None	Mild-Moderate (ie, diuretic-responsive)	Severe or Refractory
Bilirubin (mg/dL)	<2	2–3	>3
Albumin (g/dL)	>3.5	2.8–3.5	<2.8
INR	<1.7	1.7–2.3	>2.3
Operative Mortality Risk			
5–6 Points = CTP A	10%		
7–9 Points = CTP B	30%		
10–15 Points = CTP C	82%		

Adapted from Schneider PD. Preoperative assessment of liver function, Surg Clin N Am 2004;84(2):358; with permission.

Ascites

The development of ascites is the most common initial decompensating event in previously compensated patients. All patients with a new diagnosis of ascites should undergo diagnostic paracentesis. Ascitic fluid should be sent for cell count with differential, culture, fluid albumin, and fluid total protein. A cell count and differential should be sent every time a paracentesis is performed to assess for the presence of neutrocytic ascites (fluid polymorphonuclear cell count [PMN] >250/mm^3), which is used as a surrogate for the diagnosis of spontaneous bacterial peritonitis (SBP). Fluid albumin can be used to calculate a serum-ascites albumin gradient, which in combination with the fluid total protein can help to assess the etiology of ascites. A SAAG > 1.1 implies the presence of either portal hypertension or heart failure; the latter is more likely if the ascitic fluid total protein (AFTP) is > 2.5 g/dL. A SAAG < 1.1 accompanied by an AFTP > 2.5 implies a transudative process such as malignancy or tuberculosis, while a SAAG < 1.1 and AFTP < 2.5 implies the presence of nephrotic ascites.

Patients presenting with mild-to-moderate ascites are first managed with a combination of sodium restriction (<2000 mg/d) and diuretic therapy.[21] Initial diuretic therapy should include a combination of furosemide and spironolactone, at doses of 40 mg and 100 mg, respectively.[21] Doses can be increased gradually (eg, 50% increase every 3–5 days) while maintaining the 40:100 ratio to maximum doses of 160 mg and 400 mg of furosemide and spironolactone, respectively. Patients should be monitored for complications, including hypo- and hyperkalemia, hyponatremia, and renal

Table 7 Model for End-Stage Liver Disease and Model for End-Stage Liver Disease-Na score	
Scoring System	**Equation**
MELD	$0.957 \times \text{Log}_e(\text{creatinine mg/dL}) + 0.378 \times \text{Log}_e(\text{bilirubin mg/dL}) + 1.120 \times \text{Log}_e(\text{INR}) + 0.643$
MELD-Na	MELD = MELD(i) + 1.32*(137-Na) − [0.033*MELD(i)*(137-Na)] Note: Na <125 entered as 125, Na >137 entered as 137

insufficiency. Painful gynecomastia may develop with the use of spironolactone because of its partial antiandrogen effect. In this setting amiloride or eplerenone may be substituted.[22] Torsemide may be substituted for furosemide if response to furosemide is inadequate.

Among patients presenting to the hospital for the first time with tense ascites, large-volume paracentesis (LVP) is often the first step in treatment. Concurrent administration of albumin (8 g/L ascites removed) can mitigate the risk of postparacentesis hypotension and AKI. Elevated INR and thrombocytopenia do not contraindicate LVP; prophylactic transfusion of plasma and platelets prior to LVP is unnecessary unless coagulopathy is profound (INR >5, platelet count <20,000/μL, and fibrinogen <100 mg/dL).

Refractory ascites can be categorized as diuretic-resistant (unresponsive to maximum doses) or diuretic-intractable (responsive but diuresis limited by adverse effects). Once refractory ascites develop, diuretics are discontinued, and serial LVP is instituted. Peritoneal drainage catheters are not indicated because of a high risk of secondary peritonitis. Some patients with refractory ascites may be candidates for a transjugular intrahepatic portosystemic shunt (TIPS). TIPS reduces portal hypertension and has been shown to improve control of ascites (vs serial LVP) and may improve TFS. Patients must be carefully selected. Relative contraindications include but are not limited to: MELD greater than 18, age greater than 70, pulmonary hypertension, bilirubin greater than 5 mg/dL, serum creatinine greater than 3 mg/dL, portal vein thrombosis, and poorly controlled hepatic encephalopathy. Even among well-selected patients, post-TIPS hepatic encephalopathy may occur.[22]

Hepatorenal syndrome

Hepatorenal syndrome (HRS) is the development of functional renal failure in a patient with ESLD that occurs as a result of cirrhosis-induced circulatory dysfunction, RAAS activation, and renal vasoconstriction. The terms type 1- type 2-HRS are no longer used in favor of defining AKI in cirrhosis based on Kidney Disease Improving Global Outcomes (KDIGO) definition of AKI. Using these definitions, AKI is defined by the development of an increase in serum creatinine (SCr) of at least 0.3 mg/dL from baseline in 24 hours. Additional criteria necessary for the diagnosis of HRS are noted in **Table 8**. The differential diagnosis of AKI-HRS includes hypovolemia-induced AKI and acute tubular necrosis. These may be difficult to differentiate, as inciting factors (eg, infection and GI bleeding) may be common to all 3 forms of AKI. Management of HRS is summarized in **Table 8**. Treatment should be continued until SCr reaches baseline or for no more than 14 days if there is no response to treatment.[23] In patients who progress despite treatment, renal replacement therapy may be required as a bridge to LT. Patients with prolonged AKI-HRS may be candidates for simultaneous liver-kidney transplantation.

Spontaneous Bacterial Peritonitis

SBP is the most common infection seen among cirrhotic patients, occurring in up to 10% of hospitalized patients. All patients admitted to the hospital should undergo diagnostic paracentesis to assess for the presence of SBP. SBP is defined by the development of a bacterial infection in ascitic fluid without an identifiable intrabdominal source (eg, a perforation or abscess). A positive ascitic fluid culture occurs in only approximately 30% to 40% of cases of SBP, so the diagnosis is most often made based on a surrogate marker (ascites with PMN >250 cells/mm³). Patients who have culture-negative neutrocytic ascites should be managed as if they have SBP,

Table 8
Hepatorenal syndrome management

Serum Creatine Increase	Management
SCr >0.3 mg/dL (or an increase of >1.5- to twofold) from baseline to SCr <1.5 mg/dL	Diuretic withdrawal and close monitoring
SCr >1.5 mg/dL OR SCr >two- to threefold from baseline	Diuretic withdrawal Volume expansion with albumin 1 g/kg x 48 h If no response to volume expansion + meets criteria for HRS*, initiate vasoconstrictor therapy: • Midodrine 5–10 mg 3 times daily + octreotide 100 μg subcutaneously/intravenously 3 times daily or • Terlipressin 0.5–2 mg every 4–6 h • Norepinephrine 0.5–3 mg/h Vasoconstrictor therapy should be given in combination with albumin 20–40 g/d

*Criteria for HRS include AKI and: no improvement in SCr after 2 d of volume expansion and diuretic withdrawal, absence of shock, no recent use of nephrotoxic agents, and no evidence of structural renal injury (ie, no proteinuria, hematuria, or sonographic evidence of kidney disease).

Adapted from European Association for the Study of the Liver. EASL Clinical Practice Guidelines for the management of patients with decompensated cirrhosis. J Hepatol 2018;69(2):406–60; with permission.

as should patients who have non-neutrocytic bacterascites. Polymicrobial bacterascites or a very high PMN count greater than 2000/mm^3 may indicate a secondary source of infection.

Empiric antibiotic therapy for uncomplicated SBP includes the use of a third-generation cephalosporin such as cefotaxime or ceftriaxone for 5 days. In addition, intravenous albumin should be given at a dose of 1.5 g/kg at diagnosis and 1 g/kg 48h later; this protocol has been demonstrated to reduce precipitation of HRS and improve survival.[24] A repeat diagnostic paracentesis in 48 hours is helpful to assess response to treatment (ie, a reduction in fluid PMN of >25%). A lack of response may suggest the presence of an antibiotic-resistant organism and should prompt a broadening of antibiotic coverage. European guidelines recommend starting treatment with a carbapenem in patients with nosocomial SBP.[22]

Patients who survive an episode of SBP should be started on secondary prophylaxis indefinitely after initial treatment because of the high risk of recurrence (up to 70% at 1 year). Daily norfloxacin can reduce the recurrence of SBP to 20% at 1 year.[25] In the United States, ciprofloxacin is used in place of norfloxacin. Trimethoprim-sulfamethoxazole is effective in most patients who have a contraindication to quinolone therapy. Proton pump inhibitors increase the risk of SBP in cirrhotic patients and should be avoided unless there is a strong indication.[21]

Primary SBP prophylaxis is indicated in cirrhotic patients with GI bleeding, which may lead to increased translocation of gut flora and predispose to the development of SBP. A 7-day course of ceftriaxone at a dose of 1 g/d is recommended; patients can be transitioned to an oral quinolone to complete therapy as an outpatient if they are stable for discharge. Patients with a low ascitic fluid total protein less than 1.5 g/dL and renal failure (SCr >1.5 mg/dL, blood urea nitrogen [BUN] >25 mg/dL, or SNa <130 mEq/L) or liver failure (bilirubin >3 mg/dL or CTP score >9) should also receive primary prophylaxis indefinitely, as this reduces 3-month mortality and the 1-year probability of SBP (7% vs 61%).[22]

Variceal hemorrhage Gastroesophageal varices are present in up to 85% of patients with decompensated cirrhosis and develop as a direct consequence of portal hypertension. Variceal hemorrhage (VH) is among the most dramatic presentations of decompensated cirrhosis and occurs at a rate of about 10% to 15% per year. Six-week mortality following VH is 15% to 25%, and if left untreated, VH will recur in 60% at 1 year. To prevent VH, primary prophylaxis with a nonselective beta blocker (NSBB) or endoscopic variceal ligation (EVL) should be considered in patients with large varices, or in those with small high-risk varices and those with CTP-C cirrhosis.[19]

Most patients with VH present with hematemesis, although melena or hematochezia may also be noted. Patients with VH generally show signs of hemodynamic instability. Initial management of VH is similar to that of any patient with GI bleeding, with establishment of large-bore peripheral intravenous access, followed by resuscitation with crystalloid and blood. A restrictive transfusion strategy with a target hemoglobin of 7 mg/dL is recommended, as overtransfusion is deleterious and can increase portal pressures, risking continued hemorrhage. Transfusion of fresh frozen plasma (FFP) is not indicated. Patients should be intubated for airway protection if they are encephalopathic or have massive hematemesis. Initial medical therapy includes the administration of ceftriaxone for SBP prophylaxis and vasoconstrictor therapy to reduce portal inflow. Octreotide is indicated for this purpose, and has been shown to improve control of bleeding, although it does not appear to have any impact on mortality. Once VH is confirmed via endoscopy, there is no role for PPI therapy.

Endoscopy should be performed as soon as the patient is appropriately resuscitated, with EVL if esophageal varices are the likely etiology of hemorrhage. Following successful EVL, octreotide infusion is continued for a total of 5 days and antibiotics continued for 7 days. The patient can be transitioned to an NSBB once they are hemodynamically stable. Secondary prophylaxis to prevent rebleeding requires combination therapy with NSBB and serial EVL. Patients who survive an episode of VH treated with EVL need follow-up endoscopy within 2 to 4 weeks for surveillance of varices and EVL of remaining varices. EVL is performed every 2 to 4 weeks until variceal eradication, at which time surveillance endoscopy can be done in 3 months.

If bleeding cannot be controlled endoscopically, balloon tamponade may be performed, ideally by an experienced provider. Balloon tamponade is not a definitive therapy and must be followed by a more durable therapy, typically an emergent TIPS. Patients who undergo TIPS do not need to continue beta-blocker therapy or undergo follow-up endoscopy, as this procedure lowers portal pressures via structural modification to portal flow.

Gastric variceal hemorrhage is more problematic than esophageal VH, because endoscopic hemostasis is more difficult. Endoscopic options for gastric VH include EVL for varices that track along the gastric cardia and cyanoacrylate glue injection for fundic or antral varices. These patients should be evaluated for TIPS or other interventions, including balloon-occluded retrograde transvenous obliteration.[19]

Hepatic encephalopathy Hepatic encephalopathy (HE) occurs in up to 16% to 21% of patients with decompensated cirrhosis. Its presentation can be protean, ranging from minimal alterations in executive function and attention to coma.

Precipitating factors for new or worsening HE may include infection, GI bleeding, electrolyte disturbances, constipation, and portal vein thrombosis. Indolent infection is an especially common precipitant of HE, and appropriate evaluation including diagnostic paracentesis, blood, urine, and ascitic fluid culture should be performed. Alternate diagnoses should also be ruled out; patients with any focal deficits on neurologic examination should undergo brain imaging to assess for vascular or structural lesions.

Urinary toxicology is also recommended to assess for the influence of illicit substances. Measurement of arterial ammonia levels is not useful unless it is within normal limits, where an alternate diagnosis should be suspected. Intubation should be considered if patients are unable to protect their airway.

Lactulose remains the mainstay for the management of the patient with acute HE. The initial recommended dose for overt HE is 25 mL every 1 to 2 hours until 2 soft bowel movements are produced, after which the dose can be titrated to achieve 2 to 3 soft bowel movements daily. Excess bowel movements after initial improvement in HE can lead to electrolyte disturbances including hypernatremia, which may in turn worsen encephalopathy. Rifaximin is an important adjunct to lactulose that has been shown to reduce recurrence of HE and prevent readmission for overt HE among patients with prior admissions for HE.[26]

DISCLOSURE

The authors have nothing to disclose.

REFERENCES

1. Bernal W, Wendon J. Acute liver failure. N Engl J Med 2013;369(26):2525–34.
2. Roussel uclaf causality assessment method (RUCAM) in drug induced liver injury. LiverTox: clinical and research information on drug-induced liver injury. Bethesda (MD): National Institute of Diabetes and Digestive and Kidney Diseases; 2012.
3. Clinical practice guidelines panel, Wendon J, Panel members, Cordoba J, et al. EASL clinical practical guidelines on the management of acute (fulminant) liver failure. J Hepatol 2017;66(5):1047–81.
4. Chalasani N, Bonkovsky HL, Fontana R, et al. Features and outcomes of 899 patients with drug-induced liver injury: the DILIN prospective study. Gastroenterology 2015;148(7):1340–52.e7.
5. Reuben A, Tillman H, Fontana RJ, et al. Outcomes in adults with acute liver failure between 1998 and 2013: an observational cohort study. Ann Intern Med 2016; 164(11):724–32.
6. Bunchorntavakul C, Reddy KR. Acetaminophen (APAP or N-Acetyl-p-Aminophenol) and acute liver failure. Clin Liver Dis 2018;22(2):325–46.
7. Kamar N, Bendall R, Legrand-Abravanel F, et al. Hepatitis E. Lancet 2012; 379(9835):2477–88.
8. Terrault NA, Lok ASF, McMahon BJ, et al. Update on prevention, diagnosis, and treatment of chronic hepatitis B: AASLD 2018 hepatitis B guidance. Hepatology 2018;67(4):1560–99.
9. Reddy KR, Beavers KL, Hammond SP, et al. American Gastroenterological Association Institute guideline on the prevention and treatment of hepatitis B virus reactivation during immunosuppressive drug therapy. Gastroenterology 2015; 148(1):215–9, quiz e16.
10. European Association for the Study of the Liver. EASL clinical practice guidelines: autoimmune hepatitis. J Hepatol 2015;63(4):971–1004.
11. Tapper EB, Sengupta N, Bonder A. The incidence and outcomes of ischemic hepatitis: a systematic review with meta-analysis. Am J Med 2015;128(12): 1314–21.
12. Lee WM, Hynan LS, Rossaro L, et al. Intravenous N-acetylcysteine improves transplant-free survival in early stage non-acetaminophen acute liver failure. Gastroenterology 2009;137(3):856–64, 864.e1.

13. Clemmesen JO, Larsen FS, Kondrup J, et al. Cerebral herniation in patients with acute liver failure is correlated with arterial ammonia concentration. Hepatology 1999;29(3):648–53.
14. Vaquero J, Polson J, Chung C, et al. Infection and the progression of hepatic encephalopathy in acute liver failure. Gastroenterology 2003;125(3):755–64.
15. Stravitz RT, Lisman T, Luketic VA, et al. Minimal effects of acute liver injury/acute liver failure on hemostasis as assessed by thromboelastography. J Hepatol 2012; 56(1):129–36.
16. McPhail MJW, Farne H, Senvar N, et al. Ability of King's College criteria and model for end-stage liver disease scores to predict mortality of patients with acute liver failure: a meta-analysis. Clin Gastroenterol Hepatol 2016;14(4): 516–25.e5 [quiz: e43].
17. Sheikh MF, Unni N, Agarwal B. Neurological monitoring in acute liver failure. J Clin Exp Hepatol 2018;8(4):441–7.
18. D'Amico G, Garcia-Tsao G, Pagliaro L. Natural history and prognostic indicators of survival in cirrhosis: a systematic review of 118 studies. J Hepatol 2006;44(1): 217–31.
19. Garcia-Tsao G, Abraldes JG, Berzigotti A, et al. Portal hypertensive bleeding in cirrhosis: risk stratification, diagnosis, and management: 2016 practice guidance by the American Association for the study of liver diseases. Hepatology 2017; 65(1):310–35.
20. Nagai S, Chau LC, Schilke RE, et al. Effects of allocating livers for transplantation based on model for end-stage liver disease-sodium scores on patient outcomes. Gastroenterology 2018;155(5):1451–62.e3.
21. Runyon BA, AASLD. Introduction to the revised American Association for the Study of Liver Diseases practice guideline management of adult patients with ascites due to cirrhosis 2012. Hepatology 2013;57(4):1651–3.
22. European Association for the Study of the Liver. EASL clinical practice guidelines for the management of patients with decompensated cirrhosis. J Hepatol 2018; 69(2):406–60.
23. Ginès P, Solà E, Angeli P, et al. Hepatorenal syndrome. Nat Rev Dis Primers 2018; 4(1):23.
24. Sigal SH, Stanca CM, Fernandez J, et al. Restricted use of albumin for spontaneous bacterial peritonitis. Gut 2007;56(4):597–9.
25. Ginés P, Rimola A, Planas R, et al. Norfloxacin prevents spontaneous bacterial peritonitis recurrence in cirrhosis: results of a double-blind, placebo-controlled trial. Hepatology 1990;12(4):716–24.
26. Vilstrup H, Amodio P, Bajaj J, et al. Hepatic encephalopathy in chronic liver disease: 2014 practice guideline by the American Association for the Study of Liver Diseases and the European Association for the Study of the Liver. Hepatology 2014;60(2):715–35.

Catheter-Associated Urinary Tract Infection, *Clostridioides difficile* Colitis, Central Line–Associated Bloodstream Infection, and Methicillin-Resistant *Staphylococcus aureus*

Matthew Luzum, MD, MPH, Jonathan Sebolt, MD,
Vineet Chopra, MD, MSc*

KEYWORDS

- Central line–associated bloodstream infection (CLABSI)
- Catheter-associated urinary tract infection (CAUTI) • *Clostridioides difficile* colitis
- Hospital-acquired infection • Methicillin-resistant *Staphylococcus aureus*
- Bloodstream infection • Urinary tract infection

KEY POINTS

- Restricting indwelling catheter use is the most important way of preventing catheter-associated urinary tract infection (CAUTI).
- Antibiotic use is the primary risk factor for developing *Clostridioides difficile* infection.
- Treatment of initial episodes of *C difficile* depends on disease severity; treatment of recurrent episodes depends on treatment selection for the initial episode.
- Choosing the least invasive and most appropriate vascular catheter is a novel but foundational component in preventing central line–associated bloodstream infection (CLABSI).
- Appropriate management of CLABSI includes prompt collection of blood cultures, appropriate selection of empiric antimicrobial therapy, consideration of catheter removal, and deescalation of antimicrobial therapy once culture results are available.

Continued

The Division of Hospital Medicine, Department of Medicine, University of Michigan, 2800 Plymouth Road, Building 16 #432W, Ann Arbor, MI 48109, USA
* Corresponding author.
E-mail address: vineetc@umich.edu

Med Clin N Am 104 (2020) 663–679
https://doi.org/10.1016/j.mcna.2020.02.004
0025-7125/20/Published by Elsevier Inc.

medical.theclinics.com

Continued

- Methicillin-resistant *Staphylococcus aureus* (MRSA) is resistant to almost all β-lactams. It can cause skin and soft tissue infections, pneumonia, osteoarticular infections, bacteremia, and endocarditis.
- The emergence of vancomycin resistance has led to increased treatment failure in patients with MRSA infections.

CATHETER-ASSOCIATED URINARY TRACT INFECTION
Background and Epidemiology

Catheter-associated bacteriuria, which is generally reported but does not distinguish between catheter-associated asymptomatic bacteriuria (CA-ASB) and catheter-associated urinary tract infection (CAUTI), is the most common health care–associated infection worldwide. Among adult inpatient floors and long-term care facilities, incidence estimates for CAUTI range from 0.1 to 3.1 and 1.5 to 3.3 per 1000 catheter days, respectively. The use and duration of catheterization are the most important risk factors in developing CAUTI. Despite this, between 15% and 25% of patients may have a catheter placed at some point during their hospitalizations. Other risk factors for developing CAUTI include female sex, older age, and diabetes.[1,2]

Diagnosis

Among patients with an indwelling urethral or suprapubic catheter or intermittent catheterization, the diagnosis of CAUTI is defined by:

1. The presence of symptoms or signs consistent with a urinary tract infection, and
2. The absence of other identified sources of infection, and
3. At least 10^3 colony-forming units per milliliter of at least 1 bacterial species in either:
   a. A single catheter specimen, or
   b. In a midstream voided specimen from a patient whose catheter has been removed within the previous 48 hours

The signs and symptoms of CAUTI may vary depending on the patient population at risk. Typical signs and symptoms include new-onset or worsening fever, rigors, altered mentation, malaise, or lethargy with no other identified cause. The presence of flank pain, costovertebral angle tenderness, acute hematuria, and pelvic discomfort may indicate an ascending or more complex infection. Among those whose catheters have been removed within the previous 48 hours, compatible signs and symptoms of CAUTI include dysuria, urgent or frequent urination, and suprapubic pain or tenderness. Because patients with spinal cord injury have atypical symptoms, the presence of increased spasticity, autonomic dysreflexia, or a sense of unease may suggest CAUTI.

In catheterized patients, pyuria is not diagnostic of CAUTI and should not be used to differentiate between CA-ASB and CAUTI. Similarly, pyuria accompanying CA-ASB should not be interpreted as an indication for antimicrobial treatment. However, the absence of pyuria in a symptomatic patient suggests a diagnosis other than CAUTI (ie, high negative predictive value). Among catheterized patients, the presence or absence of odorous or cloudy urine alone should not be used to differentiate CA-ASB from CAUTI or as an indication for urine culture or antimicrobial therapy.[2]

Treatment

Antimicrobial therapy is recommended for all patients with symptomatic CAUTI, and the treatment is similar to that of a complicated urinary tract infection. If possible, urine cultures should always be obtained before treatment, and empiric therapy should be based on local resistance patterns. When culture results become available, empiric therapy should be narrowed to pathogen susceptibility. Among patients whose catheters have been in place for at least 2 weeks and who have continued indications for a catheter, the catheter should be replaced before initiating treatment because catheter biofilms may complicate therapy. In addition, urine cultures should be obtained from freshly replaced catheters to obtain more accurate culture results. If catheter use is no longer indicated, obtain a voided midstream urine sample for culture.

Among patients who have quick symptom resolution, the standard duration of therapy for CAUTI is 7 days, and patients with a delayed response should be treated for 10 to 14 days regardless of whether catheter use continues. Women aged less than or equal to 65 years without upper urinary tract symptoms may complete a 3-day treatment course after the urinary catheter is removed. Among patients with a fungal CAUTI, guidelines strongly recommend removing the indwelling catheter.

Insertion and maintenance of catheters should be performed by trained personnel following strict aseptic technique with a closed drainage system. In all patients, indwelling urinary catheters should be removed as early as possible. Routine replacement of catheters is not recommended; however, mechanical problems such as bladder outlet obstruction may require catheter reinsertion if these remain uncorrected. Condom catheters may improve patient comfort, but whether they are preferable to short-term or long-term indwelling catheterization for reduction of CAUTI is uncertain.[2]

Disease Complications and Prognosis

CAUTIs have implications for patients and health systems. Health care–associated urinary tract infections may extend hospital stay by 2 to 4 days. Complications associated with CAUTI include acute pyelonephritis, periurethral abscess, bacteremia or sepsis, prostatitis, and epididymo-orchitis. More broadly, genitourinary infections are responsible for approximately 15% of hospital-acquired bacteremia, and the mortality of nosocomial bacteremia caused by urinary tract infection is about 13%. Specifically, catheter-associated bacteriuria is complicated by bacteremia in less than 1% to 4% of cases. Although the exact relationship between catheter-associated bacteriuria and mortality is uncertain, the populations at highest risk of mortality include women, elderly patients, and immunosuppressed patients.[2,3]

Prevention Strategies

Despite being recognized as one of the first hospital-acquired conditions selected for nonpayment by Medicare in 2008 and later classified as a never event, CAUTI prevention has remained challenging for several reasons. An emphasis on technological interventions, a dearth of randomized controlled trials, and multicomponent interventions remain some of the challenges in facilitating CAUTI prevention. These limitations have resulted in guideline recommendations based on low to moderate quality of evidence. In addition, monitoring catheter use and CAUTI rates and implementing CAUTI interventions is resource intensive, and interventions designed to limit catheters requires changing habits of patients and providers.

Recognizing these challenges, the Centers for Disease Control–funded States Targeting Reduction in Infections via Engagement (STRIVE) initiative used recent literature reviews, guidelines, and the collective experience of a multidisciplinary team to develop a tiered approach to CAUTI prevention based on cost, level of evidence, and expected magnitude of an intervention's effect.[4,5] The first tier of STRIVE recommendations, which emphasize interventions that are cost-effective and have greater effect, consists of standardizing basic supplies, procedures, and processes to avoid unnecessary testing and disrupt the life cycle of urinary catheters at certain steps. First-tier interventions emphasize placing urinary catheters for appropriate reasons (**Box 1**), encouraging use of alternatives to indwelling catheters, ensuring proper aseptic insertion technique and maintenance procedures, optimizing prompt removal of unneeded catheters, and obtaining urine cultures only if patients have symptoms of a urinary tract infection. Catheter replacement restrictions and urinary retention protocols, which are directed toward avoiding unnecessary catheter placement, have been shown to reduce the use of catheters, decrease the proportion of catheters in place without a physician order, and decrease the proportion of catheters in place without an appropriate indication. Other interventions, such as urinary catheter reminder systems and automatic stop orders to prompt catheter removal, have been effective in reducing duration of urinary catheterization and CAUTI in hospitalized adults.[5] The STRIVE team recommended hospitals implement, review, and audit compliance with each first-tier intervention before moving on to a second tier of enhanced practices.[4]

If CAUTI rates remain increased after implementing first-tier interventions, STRIVE recommended hospitals perform a self-assessment using the CAUTI guide to patient safety (GPS) and the targeted assessment for prevention (TAP) tool. The CAUTI GPS is a validated needs-assessment survey that can provide additional guidance for prevention (available at https://www.catheterout.org/cauti-gps.html). The CAUTI TAP tool helps identify resources for addressing prevention gaps and consists of identifying units with higher than expected CAUTI rates, administering TAP assessment tools to identify prevention gaps by location, and accessing prevention resources to address identified gaps. After starting with a needs assessment using CAUTI GPS

Box 1
Examples of indications for indwelling urethral catheter use

Appropriate indications for indwelling urinary catheters
- Acute urinary retention or bladder outlet obstruction
- Need for accurate measurements of urinary output in critically ill patients
- Perioperative use for selected surgical procedures
  - Urologic or other surgery on contiguous structures of genitourinary tract
  - Anticipated prolonged surgery duration (catheters inserted for this reason should be removed in postanesthesia care unit)
  - Patients anticipated to receive large-volume infusions or diuretics during surgery
  - Need for intraoperative monitoring of urinary output
- To assist in healing of open sacral or perineal wounds in incontinent patients
- Prolonged immobilization (eg, potentially unstable thoracic or lumbar spine, pelvic fractures)
- Improve comfort for end-of-life care as needed

Inappropriate indications for indwelling catheters
- A substitute for nursing care of the patient or resident with incontinence
- A means to obtain urine for culture or other diagnostic tests when the patient can voluntarily void
- Prolonged postoperative duration without appropriate indications (eg, structural repair of urethra or contiguous structures, prolonged effect of epidural anesthesia)

and TAP, additional second-tier interventions include performing catheter rounds with targeted education to optimize appropriate use, providing real-time feedback to front-line staff about infection and catheter use; observing and documenting competency of catheter insertion, and performing root cause analyses or focused reviews of identified infections.[4]

CLOSTRIDIOIDES DIFFICILE COLITIS
Background and Epidemiology

Clostridioides difficile (previously classified as *Clostridium difficile*) is a spore-forming, toxin-producing anaerobic bacterium that may colonize or infect the colon to cause invasive colitis. *C difficile* colitis is one of the most common causes of hospital-acquired diarrhea. Clinical manifestations of *C difficile* infection range from an asymptomatic carrier state to mild diarrhea or fulminant and life-threatening colitis. Transmission of spores occurs from person to person via the fecal-oral route, and spores can survive on dry inanimate surfaces for up to 5 months. Antibiotic use alters the normal colonic flora and is the primary risk factor for clinical infection. Although the risk of invasive disease varies by antibiotic class, nearly every antibiotic has been associated or suspected to clinically manifest *C difficile* infection. Beyond antibiotic use, other major risk factors for invasive disease include age greater than 64 years, severe illness, recent or current hospitalization, duration of hospitalization, human immunodeficiency virus infection, and stomach acid–suppressing medications.[6]

The prevalence of colonization with *C difficile* is estimated to be 7% to 26% and 5% to 7% in acute care and long-term care settings, respectively. The global estimated cumulative incidence for all ages of *C difficile* infection is 49.36 per 100,000 population per year with overall incidence rates of 2.24 per 1000 admissions per year and 3.54 per 10,000 patient-days.[7] In the United States, the hospitalization rates per 100,000 population increased from 48.8 to 114.6 between 1996 and 2008, and the highest estimated cumulative incidence occurred in the elderly (323.32 per 100,000 population per year).[7] Similarly, among hospitalized patients between 2001 and 2010, the incidence of *C difficile* infection almost doubled (4.5–8.2 cases per 1000 discharges, respectively), and it has become the most common causative pathogen of health care–associated infections.[8]

Diagnosis

Traditional risk factors for *C difficile* infection are antibiotic exposure, hospitalization, and increasing age. Exposure to systemic antibiotics disrupts the microbiome and increases the risk of *C difficile* infection 2-fold to 16-fold. Similarly, in patients who receive concomitant systemic antibiotics while being treated for *C difficile* infection, the time to resolution of diarrhea is longer, cure rate is lower, and episodes of recurrence are greater. The risk of *C difficile* infection increases proportionally with the length of hospital stay, longer duration of systemic antibiotics, and number of antibiotics used. Other established and emerging risk factors, such as use of proton pump inhibitors, are listed in **Box 2**.[9]

The most common presenting symptom is diarrhea. Importantly, fulminant colitis may present with severe abdominal pain or colonic distension, and diarrhea may be absent because of bowel ileus. Patients should be evaluated for signs of systemic illness, such as fever, tachycardia, and hypotension. Serial abdominal examinations assessing for tenderness, increasing distension, diminished bowel sounds, and peritoneal signs should be performed. Stool testing options include enzyme immunoassays for *C difficile* toxins, polymerase chain reaction, stool glutamate

> **Box 2**
> **Risk factors for *Clostridioides difficile* infection**
>
> - Age greater than 65 years
> - Previous hospitalization and prolonged length of stay
> - Nursing home or long-term care facility residence
> - Contact with active carriers
> - Antibiotic exposure (increased risk with prolonged use or multiple antibiotics)
> - Consumption of processed meat
> - Previous gastrointestinal surgery or endoscopy
> - Comorbid conditions
> - Malignancy and chemotherapy
> - Cystic fibrosis
> - Diabetes mellitus
> - Cirrhosis
> - Chronic kidney disease
> - Inflammatory bowel disease
> - Immunosuppression, immunodeficiency, or human immunodeficiency virus
> - Malnutrition
> - Hypoalbuminemia
> - Use of proton pump inhibitors
> - Solid organ or hematopoietic stem cell transplant
> - Presence of gastrostomy or jejunostomy tube
>
> *Adapted from* Khanna S, Pardi DS. Clostridium difficile infection: new insights into management. Mayo Clin Proc 2012;87(11):1108; with permission.

dehydrogenase (GDH) assay, and toxigenic culture and cell culture cytotoxicity. Disease severity is stratified by white blood cell count; serum creatinine level; and the presence or absence of hypotension or shock, ileus, or megacolon.[10]

The diagnosis of *C difficile* colitis is based on a combination of clinical and laboratory findings. The primary symptom of *C difficile* is diarrhea, defined as at least 3 unformed stools within a 24-hour period. Laboratory findings include either positive stool testing for *C difficile* toxin, or colonoscopic or biopsy findings consistent with pseudomembranous colitis. Because testing can detect asymptomatic carrier states, patients with unexplained and new-onset diarrhea in the appropriate clinical context (eg, recently exposed to antibiotics) are ideal targets for stool tests. Currently available options include GDH assays, enzyme immunoassays that detect toxins A or B, nucleic acid amplification tests (NAAT), and cell culture cytotoxicity assays or toxigenic cultures.

Among institutions without previously agreed-on criteria for stool submission, the Infectious Disease Society of America (IDSA) and Society for Healthcare Epidemiology of America (SHEA) guideline suggests a multistep algorithm instead of using NAAT alone. Criteria should include only submitting stool specimens from patients with at least 3 unexplained, new-onset, and unformed stools in 24 hours. Patients who have received laxatives or who may have other causes for loose stools (eg, recent exposure to oral contrast or tube feeds) should not be tested. Examples of multistep algorithms include a GDH plus toxin assay, a GDH plus toxin assay arbitrated by NAAT, and NAAT plus a toxin assay. Among institutions with previously agreed-on criteria for stool submission, either NAAT alone or a multistep algorithm is recommended.[10]

Assessing and quantifying disease severity is important for choosing a treatment approach. In patients with severe symptoms, computed tomography to evaluate for complications such as severe colitis, megacolon, or ileus may be appropriate. The IDSA/SHEA guideline categorizes *C difficile* disease as nonsevere, severe, or fulminant.

Treatment

Asymptomatic carriers do not need treatment. For symptomatic adults, carefully review antibiotic use and discontinue unnecessary treatment whenever possible. If continued antibiotic therapy is warranted, deescalation to a narrow-spectrum antibiotic for the shortest possible duration is recommended. The treatment of initial and recurrent disease is summarized in.[10]

In all cases, antimotility agents (including antiperistaltic and narcotic medications) should be reduced or discontinued.[9] Hospitalized patients should be placed in contact precautions (gown and gloves) to prevent spore transmission. Hand hygiene with soap and water is preferred to alcohol-based products before and after contact with a patient with *C difficile* infection, after removing gloves, and after direct contact with feces or an area with likely fecal contamination. However, in routine or endemic settings, hand hygiene may be performed with either soap and water or an alcohol-based product.[10]

Surgical consultation should be considered if imaging suggests perforation or toxic megacolon, or severe illness develops despite treatment. A leukocyte count greater than or equal to 25,000 cell/mL or lactate level greater than or equal to 5 mmol/L has been associated with high mortality and these may be indicators for early surgery. If surgical management is necessary for patients who are severely ill, guidelines recommend performing a subtotal colectomy and preserving the rectum. An alternative approach is performing a diverting loop ileostomy with colonic lavage followed by antegrade vancomycin flushes. All patients should be monitored for reduction in stool frequency, improvement in stool consistency, normalization of abdominal findings, hydration, and resolution of leukocytosis.

Disease Complications and Prognosis

Complications of severe *C difficile* infection include toxic megacolon, ileus, bowel perforation, dehydration, acidosis, peritonitis, electrolyte imbalances, hypoalbuminemia, hypotension, renal failure, sepsis and septic shock, and death. Among patients with hospital-acquired *C difficile* infection, the absolute risk of death is 10%.[11] Traditional surgical approaches, such as subtotal or total colectomy, have mortalities as high as 50%. Variables associated with increased mortality include older age, chronic comorbidities, binary toxin genes (polymerase chain reaction [PCR] ribotypes 014, 015, 018, 027, 056, and 027), and renal impairment.[9] Disease recurrence has been reported in 10% to 30% of patients.[10] Up to 25% of patients have their first recurrence within 30 days after completing treatment; risk factors for recurrence include older age, severity of initial infection, antibiotic exposure during follow-up period, use of proton pump inhibitors, and renal insufficiency.[11]

Prevention

The STRIVE initiative recommended a standardized approach to reduce *C difficile* infections. In addition to horizontal infection prevention practices (those that are broadly applicable to several hospital-acquired infections [HAIs]), a tiered approach that grouped interventions by quality of evidence, effect size, and ease of implementation was developed. The first STRIVE tier emphasized standardization of supplies, procedures, and processes, including implementing *C difficile* infection–specific antimicrobial stewardship interventions, conducting early and appropriate *C difficile* infection testing and alerting staff of patients' infection status, preventing disease transmission using strict hand hygiene and glove use, promptly initiating and maintaining contact precautions for affected patients when they test positive and for the duration of their illness, cleaning and disinfecting the equipment and environment of affected patients, and monitoring and sharing health care–associated *C difficile* infection rates with staff and leadership.[8]

Second-tier recommendations included more capital-intense interventions that focused on personnel and resources. They include performing a needs assessment using either a GPS or TAP to tailor resources with self-identified gaps in *C difficile* infection prevention practices; extending the use of contact precautions by initiating them for symptomatic patients while testing results are pending and maintaining them until discharge (as opposed to only when affected patients become asymptomatic); implementing environmental cleaning process tools such as audit checklists and an Environmental Protection Agency sporicidal agent; and real-time feedback on hand hygiene performance with hand hygiene provider champions, competency-based training, and patient education.[8]

Preserving the intestinal microbiota is crucial to preventing *C difficile* infection. Antimicrobial stewardship, therefore, is the cornerstone of prevention. In institutional settings, prevention of transmission across patients by enforcement of contact precautions, patient isolation, and hand washing using soap and water is essential. There are insufficient data to make specific recommendations regarding the role of probiotics in prevention of primary *C difficile* infection.[10]

CENTRAL LINE–ASSOCIATED BLOODSTREAM INFECTION
Background and Epidemiology

Central line–associated bloodstream infection (CLABSI) is a preventable HAI that is associated with increased cost, morbidity, and mortality.[12–14] CLABSI is surveillance term that typifies patients with a central venous catheter (CVC) who develop a bloodstream infection (BSI) that is not attributable to another source after a focused clinical review.[15] Furthermore, the pathogen isolated must be from a single blood culture (for organisms that are not commonly present on skin) or 2 or more blood cultures (for organisms commonly present on the skin) in a patient with signs and symptoms of infection who has a central line in place at the time of the identification of the infection or within 48 hours of diagnosis.[16,17] In contrast, catheter-related bloodstream infection (CRBSI) is a clinical definition that requires (1) isolation of the same organism from the catheter, peripheral blood, or catheter tip; (2) simultaneous quantitative blood cultures with a ratio of 5:1 or higher of those from the indwelling CVC compared with peripheral blood; or (3) a differential time to positivity of CVC-derived versus peripheral blood culture positivity of more than 2 hours.[18]

CLABSI can occur via several routes; pathogenesis depends on the type of catheter and dwell time. For nontunneled catheters that have been in place for 7 days or less, infection is often related to insertion and occurs as a result of extraluminal contamination (eg, skin pathogens at the insertion site). For devices in place 8 days or more, infection likely originates from the catheter hub and endoluminal surface and is often related to maintenance. Less commonly, infection can occur via hematogenous seeding or contaminated infusates. Once contamination occurs, microbes adhere to the catheter surface and proliferate to form biofilm, which can make treatment of infection difficult (often necessitating catheter removal).

Diagnosis

Diagnosis of CLABSI requires a timely and methodical approach to reduce morbidity and mortality. If suspected, blood cultures should be drawn with prompt initiation of empiric antimicrobial therapy. Cultures should be drawn from peripheral veins as well as from CVCs in place at the time of evaluation. Given CRBSI carries a more rigorous definition, methods to accurately diagnose CRBSI include:

1. Catheter segment culture (distal 5 cm of the removed catheter tip sent for roll-plate analysis),[19]
2. Paired quantitative blood cultures, and
3. Differential time to positivity

   Identification of risk factors associated with CLABSI has been instrumental in guiding prevention efforts. Established risk factors are outlined in **Box 3**.

Treatment

If CLABSI is suspected, empiric therapy should be administered after cultures are collected. In general, the choice of empiric therapy should be tailored to:

1. Most likely causative pathogen
2. Type of catheter
3. Host characteristics
4. Local susceptibility patterns
5. Clinical stability of the patient, and
6. Presence of complications[20]

Box 3
Risk factors for central line–associated bloodstream infection

- Lengthy hospitalization before catheterization
- Prolonged duration of catheterization
- Use of multilumen catheters
- Heavy microbial colonization at the insertion site
- Heavy microbial colonization of the catheter hub
- Femoral or internal jugular vein insertion (rather than subclavian vein)
- Operator inexperience or lack of implementation of best practices during CVC insertion
- Presence of neutropenia
- Total parenteral nutrition through the catheter
- Inadequate care/maintenance of the CVC after insertion
- Type of CVC

Table 1 outlines the 2009 IDSA clinical practice guidelines for management of intravascular catheter-related infections. In addition to empiric antibiotic coverage, consideration should be given to catheter removal. Long-term catheters should be removed from patients if any of the following exist: severe sepsis; suppurative thrombophlebitis; endocarditis; BSI that continues despite more than 72 hours of appropriate antimicrobial therapy; or infections caused by *Staphylococcus aureus*, *Pseudomonas aeruginosa*, fungi, or mycobacteria. Short-term catheters should be removed from patients with infection caused by gram-negative bacilli, *S aureus*, enterococci, fungi, and mycobacteria.

Prevention

Although great progress has recently been achieved in the prevention of CLABSI, (with an observed 50% reduction in CLABSIs from 2008 to 2014 in acute care hospitals in the United States), many patients continue to experience this HAI annually.[21] Prevention of CLABSI requires a multifaceted approach with various interventions formulated around the pathophysiology of CLABSI. Progress in reducing CLABSI relates to several elements, including evidence-based checklists for catheter insertion; improved efficacy of modern skin antiseptics, such as alcohol-containing chlorhexidine; and greater awareness of risk factors, leading to focused efforts directed at the problem. The concept of a standardized approach as exemplified by a catheter bundle is now being used to improve insertion of catheters to reduce CLABSI risk.

Table 1
Empiric antimicrobial recommendations

Coverage	Patient Population	Antimicrobials
Gram positive	Patients in health care settings with increased prevalence of MRSA	IV vancomycin or daptomycin
Gram-negative bacilli	• Neutropenia • Critical illness • Femoral catheter-related BSI	Consider a fourth-generation cephalosporin, β-lactam/β-lactamase inhibitor combination, or carbapenem, with or without aminoglycoside Should be based on local antimicrobial susceptibility patterns
MDR organisms	• Neutropenia • Severely ill patients with sepsis • Known colonization with MDR organisms	Combination therapy with 2 different classes of antimicrobials against MDR gram-negative bacilli
Fungal	Sepsis with any of the following: • Total parenteral nutrition • Prolonged broad-spectrum antibiotic use • Hematologic malignancy • Solid organ or bone marrow transplant • Femoral catheter-related BSI • *Candida* colonization at multiple sites	Echinocandin

Abbreviations: IV, intravenous; MDR, multidrug resistant; MRSA, methicillin-resistant *Staphylococcus aureus*.

The CDC STRIVE project outlined a rubric for CLABSI reduction efforts. Tier 1 begins with assessment of appropriateness of vascular catheter use before placement. STRIVE recommends using the Michigan Appropriateness Guide for Intravenous Catheters (MAGIC) as an algorithmic, evidence-based guide to selecting a vascular catheter. Intervention 2 advises careful site selection and avoidance of the femoral vein for CVC placement. Intervention 3 focuses on insertion using evidence-based checklists and bundles. Intervention 4 targets care and maintenance of catheters via use of transparent, semipermeable dressings to cover the catheter site; minimizing dressing disruption; use of chlorhexidine-impregnated sponge dressings for short-term CVCs; use of the fewest device lumens; disinfecting of access ports before and after use; dressing changes every 5 to 7 days for nontunneled CVCs; and emphasis on hand hygiene and sterile insertion technique. Intervention 5 emphasizes strategies to ensure removal of unnecessary CVCs, given that decreasing dwell time decreases risk for CLABSI.

METHICILLIN-RESISTANT *STAPHYLOCOCCUS AUREUS*
Background and Epidemiology

S aureus is a gram-positive, nonmotile, coagulase-positive coccus that is both a human commensal and a cause of clinically important infections. It is found in the commensal microbiota of the nasal mucosa in 20% to 40% of the general population. Methicillin-resistant *S aureus* (MRSA) refers to a strain resistant to methicillin and almost all β-lactams, including antistaphylococcal penicillins. MRSA infections are associated with significant morbidity and mortality.[22,23]

MRSA as a pathogen was first reported in the 1960s after the introduction of methicillin, a semisynthetic β-lactam introduced in the United Kingdom in 1959 in response to penicillin resistance associated with the acquisition of a β-lactamase enzyme, *blaZ*, by *S aureus*.[24] In the decade following its initial description, MRSA was responsible for hospital outbreaks (health care–associated MRSA) in many parts of the world.[25] It has since been detected in individuals without previous health-care contact (community-associated MRSA) as well as with livestock exposure (livestock-associated MRSA). Recent data from the National Healthcare Safety Network (NHSN) report that, from 2009 to 2010, a significant percentage of *S aureus* isolates in CLABSI (54.6%), ventilator-associated pneumonia (48.4%), CAUTI (58.7%), and surgical site infections (43.7%) were methicillin resistant.[26,27] Therefore, MRSA is an important pathogen in the development of many HAIs.

Although multiple body sites can be colonized with MRSA in human beings, the anterior nares of the nose are the most frequent carriage site for *S aureus*.[28] In most cases, *S aureus* colonization precedes infection. One study of persons in whom MRSA colonization had been identified during a previous hospital stay reported that the risk of developing an MRSA infection within 18 months of detection of MRSA colonization was 29%.[29] Less commonly, infection can occur in the absence of known colonization; for example, as a result of contamination of catheters or wounds from suboptimal infection control practices.[30] MRSA preys on the sickest of patients; therefore, risk factors for MRSA colonization include severe underlying illness or comorbid conditions, prolonged hospital stay, exposure to broad-spectrum antimicrobials, presence of invasive devices (eg, CVCs), and frequent contact with the health care system or health care personnel.[31] Longitudinal studies have identified 3 temporal patterns of *S aureus* (including both methicillin-sensitive *S aureus* and MRSA) colonization. These patterns include continuous *S aureus* colonization (found in ∼15% of individuals, known as persistent carriers), intermittent colonization (present in 70% of individuals), and noncarriers (*S aureus* was never detected in 15% of individuals).[32]

Diagnosis

MRSA infections include skin and soft tissue infections, pneumonia, osteoarticular infections, bacteremia, and endocarditis. The pathogen is capable of producing numerous toxins, which can result in diverse clinical syndromes. For example, MRSA cytotoxin can induce proinflammatory changes that clinically manifest as sepsis, or enterotoxin, which can lead to toxic shock syndrome and food poisoning. In addition, MRSA-related exfoliative toxins lead to skin erythema and separation seen in staphylococcal scalded skin syndrome. Thus, a high degree of suspicion for MRSA infection should exist when dealing with virtually any presentation or body system in hospitalized settings.

Treatment

In addition to timely diagnosis of infection, prompt initiation of appropriate antibiotics for MRSA is paramount. Kumar and colleagues[33] found that, in patients with septic shock related to MRSA bacteremia, each hour of delay of appropriate antibiotic therapy was associated with increased mortality. Empiric therapy should include an antibiotic effective against MRSA and target those with risk factors for MRSA as well as those with suspected staphylococcal infection in settings known to have high rates of MRSA prevalence. Antibiotic choice, route, and duration should be tailored to the site and severity of infection and adjusted based on culture and susceptibilities. **Table 2** outlines management recommendations for common MRSA infections.

Complications and Prognosis

Since MRSA emerged as a significant nosocomial pathogen in the United States, intravenous vancomycin has been the cornerstone of therapy. However, over the years, MRSA has acquired resistance to vancomycin. Vancomycin intermediate-resistance *S aureus* first appeared in Japan in 1997 and has since been identified worldwide.[40] Vancomycin-resistant *S aureus*, first identified in Detroit, Michigan, in 2002, has a very high minimum inhibitory concentration (MIC) (>32 µg/mL) with resistance mediated by the *vanA* gene, which is thought to have been transferred from *Enterococcus faecalis* on the plasmid-borne transposon Tn1546.[41] Studies show increased clinical failure of vancomycin therapy in MRSA infections in which the isolates have increased MICs but are still susceptible. Furthermore, treatment with vancomycin in the previous 30 days is predictive of a higher MIC and lower therapeutic efficacy of vancomycin.[42–44]

Prevention

To reduce MRSA infections in acute care settings, several evidence-based infection prevention strategies have been recommended. Surveillance studies show significant reductions in hospital-onset MRSA BSIs in US hospitals and intensive care units following implementation of these strategies. Despite this progress, many US hospitals continue to experience higher than expected rates of hospital-onset MRSA infection. The STRIVE project outlined 2 tiers for MRSA prevention, with tier 1 strategies including 6 specific interventions.[45] Intervention 1 was a risk assessment strategy to determine MRSA infection burden and transmission risk. Intervention 2 focused on case reviews of each National Healthcare Safety Network–defined case of hospital-onset MRSA bacteremia so as to identify patient-level and population-level risk factors. Intervention 3 asked hospitals to establish a program to identify and track

Table 2
Management of common infections caused by methicillin-resistant *Staphylococcus aureus*

Clinical Condition	Management Recommendations
Soft tissue abscess	Surgical debridement and drainage is the mainstay of therapy Antibiotic therapy is recommended for abscesses associated with: • Severe or extensive disease • Rapid progression in presence of associated cellulitis • Signs/symptoms of systemic illness • Comorbidities or immunosuppression • Extremes of age • Abscess in an area difficult to drain • Associated septic phlebitis • Lack of response to incision and drainage alone
Skin and soft tissue infection (complicated) • Deeper soft tissue infections • Surgical/traumatic wound infection • Major abscesses • Cellulitis • Infected ulcers and burns	Empiric therapy for MRSA is recommended pending cultures Empiric treatment options include vancomycin, linezolid, daptomycin, telavancin, or clindamycin
Uncomplicated bacteremia (positive blood culture results and all of the following) • Exclusion of endocarditis • No implanted prostheses • Clearance of blood cultures drawn 2–4 d after initial set • Defervescence within 72 h of initiating effective therapy • No evidence of metastatic sites of infection	IV vancomycin or IV daptomycin recommended for at least 2 wk For complicated bacteremia, 4–6 wk of therapy is recommended, depending on the extent of infection. Infectious disease consultation is recommended in all cases of MRSA bacteremia
Infective endocarditis (native valve)	IV vancomycin or IV daptomycin for 6 wk is recommended; however, a recent trial showed that, in clinically stable patients with endocarditis on the left side of the heart (caused by *S aureus*) and adequate response to initial treatment, a shift from initial IV to oral antibiotic treatment was noninferior to continued IV antibiotic treatment Evaluation for valve replacement surgery is recommended if any of the following: • Large vegetation >10 mm in diameter • Embolic event during the first 2 wk of therapy • Severe valvular insufficiency • Valvular perforation or dehiscence • Decompensated heart failure • Perivalvular or myocardial abscess • New heart block • Persistent fevers or bacteremia
Infective endocarditis (prosthetic valve)	IV vancomycin plus PO/IV rifampin for at least 6 wk plus IV gentamicin for 2 wk Recommend early evaluation for valve replacement surgery

(continued on next page)

Table 2
(continued)

Clinical Condition	Management Recommendations
Community-acquired pneumonia	Recommend empiric MRSA coverage only if locally validated risk factors are present. Empiric treatment options include IV vancomycin or linezolid Deescalation or confirmation of need for continued therapy should be guided by cultures and nasal PCR
Hospital-acquired pneumonia/ ventilator-associated pneumonia	Empiric therapy should include MRSA coverage if any of the following: • Risk factors for antimicrobial resistance present • Units where >10%–20% of S aureus is MRSA • Units where prevalence of MRSA is unknown Empiric treatment options include IV vancomycin or linezolid Recommend a 7-d course of therapy with shorter or longer duration depending on rate of improvement of clinical, radiologic, and laboratory parameters
Osteomyelitis	Surgical debridement and drainage of associated soft tissue abscesses is mainstay of therapy Optimal route of administration of antibiotic therapy has not been established.[24] Recent OVIVA trial showed oral antibiotic therapy to be noninferior to IV therapy when used during the first 6 wk of treatment of bone and joint infection Parenteral options include vancomycin and daptomycin. TMP/SMX, linezolid, and clindamycin are available in both parenteral and oral routes
Septic arthritis	Drainage or debridement of the joint space should always be performed For antibiotic recommendations, refer to management of osteomyelitis
Health care–associated ventriculitis and meningitis	IV vancomycin is recommended empirically and as first-line therapy for confirmed MRSA, with consideration for an alternative agent if the vancomycin MIC ≥ 1 μg/mL Alternatives: linezolid, daptomycin, or TMP-SMX with selection guided by in vitro susceptibility testing Duration of treatment: 10–14 d For CNS shunt infection, shunt removal is recommended, and should not be replaced until 10 d after CSF cultures are negative

Abbreviations: CNS, central nervous system; CSF, cerebrospinal fluid; MIC, minimum inhibitory concentration; OVIVA, oral versus intravenous antibiotics; PO, by mouth; TMP/SMX, trimethoprim/sulfamethoxazole.
Data from Refs.[34–39]

patients in whom MRSA has been identified. Intervention 4 recommended the promotion and monitoring of hand hygiene compliance before and after patient contact. Intervention 5 focused on initiation of contact precautions for patients colonized or infected with MRSA. Intervention 6 recommended routine and thorough environmental cleaning of patient rooms and patient care equipment, focusing on high-touch environmental surfaces on a daily basis, when spills occur, when there is visible contamination, and at the time of discharge. These measures reduce opportunities for contamination of health care worker hands and the risk for MRSA acquisition by subsequent occupants.

CONFLICTS OF INTEREST

None declared for all coauthors. Dr V Chopra is supported by grants from the VA National Center for Patient Safety, Health Services Research and Development and the Agency for Healthcare Research and Quality.

REFERENCES

1. Hollenbeak CS, Schilling AL. The attributable cost of catheter-associated urinary tract infections in the United States: a systematic review. Am J Infect Control 2018;46(7):751–7.
2. Hooton TM, Bradley SF, Cardenas DD, et al. Diagnosis, prevention, and treatment of catheter-associated urinary tract infection in adults: 2009 International Clinical Practice Guidelines from the Infectious Diseases Society of America. Clin Infect Dis 2010;50(5):625–63.
3. Gould CV, Umscheid CA, Agarwal RK, et al. Guideline for prevention of catheter-associated urinary tract infections 2009. Infect Control Hosp Epidemiol 2010; 31(4):319–26.
4. Meddings J, Manojlovich M, Fowler KE, et al. A tiered approach for preventing catheter-associated urinary tract infection. Ann Intern Med 2019; 171(7_Supplement):S30–7.
5. Shekelle PG, Wachter RM, Pronovost PJ, et al. Making health care safer II: an updated critical analysis of the evidence for patient safety practices. Evid Rep Technol Assess (Full Rep) 2013;(211):1–945.
6. Cohen SH, Gerding DN, Johnson S, et al. Clinical practice guidelines for Clostridium difficile infection in adults: 2010 update by the society for healthcare epidemiology of America (SHEA) and the infectious diseases society of America (IDSA). Infect Control Hosp Epidemiol 2010;31(5):431–55.
7. Balsells E, Shi T, Leese C, et al. Global burden of Clostridium difficile infections: a systematic review and meta-analysis. J Glob Health 2019;9(1):010407.
8. Rohde JM, Jones K, Padron N, et al. A tiered approach for preventing Clostridioides difficile infection. Ann Intern Med 2019;171(7_Supplement):S45–51.
9. Khanna S, Pardi DS. Clostridium difficile infection: new insights into management. Mayo Clin Proc 2012;87(11):1106–17.
10. McDonald LC, Gerding DN, Johnson S, et al. Clinical practice guidelines for Clostridium difficile infection in adults and children: 2017 update by the Infectious Diseases Society of America (IDSA) and Society for Healthcare Epidemiology of America (SHEA). Clin Infect Dis 2018;66(7):987–94.
11. Deshpande A, Pasupuleti V, Thota P, et al. Risk factors for recurrent Clostridium difficile infection: a systematic review and meta-analysis. Infect Control Hosp Epidemiol 2015;36(4):452–60.

12. Umscheid CA, Mitchell MD, Doshi JA, et al. Estimating the proportion of healthcare-associated infections that are reasonably preventable and the related mortality and costs. Infect Control Hosp Epidemiol 2011;32:101–14.
13. Siempos IL, Kopterides P, Tsangaris I, et al. Impact of catheter-related bloodstream infections on the mortality of critically ill patients: a meta-analysis. Crit Care Med 2009;37:2283–9.
14. Wenzel RP, Edmond MB. The impact of hospital-acquired bloodstream infections. Emerg Infect Dis 2001;7(2):174–7.
15. Centers for Disease Control and Prevention. National healthcare safety network (NHSN) patient safety component manual. Chapter 4: Bloodstream infection event (central line-associated bloodstream infection and non-central line associated bloodstream infection). 2018. Available at: https://www.cdc.gov/nhsn/pdfs/pscmanual/pcsmanualcurrent/pdf. Accessed October 13, 2019.
16. Centers for Disease Control and Prevention (CDC). Vital signs: central line-associated blood stream infections-United States, 2001, 2008, and 2009. MMWR Morb Mortal Wkly Rep 2011;60(8):243–8.
17. Horan TC, Andrus M, Dudeck MA. CDC/NHSN surveillance definition of health care-associated infection and criteria for specific types of infections in the acute care setting. Am J Infect Control 2008;36:309–32.
18. Mermel LA, Allon M, Bouza E, et al. Clinical practice guidelines for the diagnosis and management of intravascular catheter-related infection: 2009 Update by the Infectious Diseases Society of America. Clin Infect Dis 2009;49(1):1–45.
19. Maki D, Weise C, Sarafin H. A semiquantitative culture method for identifying intravenous-catheter-related infection. N Engl J Med 1977;296:1305–9.
20. Rupp ME, Karnatak R. Intravascular catheter-related bloodstream infections. Infect Dis Clin North Am 2018;32:765–87.
21. Patel PK, Olmsted RN, Hung L, et al. A tiered approach for preventing central line-associated bloodstream infection. Ann Intern Med 2019;171(7_Supplement):S16–22.
22. Lowy F. Staphylococcus aureus infections. N Engl J Med 1998;339:520–32.
23. Wertheim HF, Melles DC, Vos MC, et al. The role of nasal carriage in Staphylococcus aureus infections. Lancet Infect Dis 2005;5:751–62.
24. Knox R. A new penicillin (BRL 1241) active against penicillin-resistant staphylococci. Br Med J 1960;2:690–3.
25. Chambers HF, Deleo FR. Waves of resistance: Staphylococcus aureus in the antibiotic era. Nat Rev Microbiol 2009;7:629–41.
26. Sievert DM, Ricks P, Edwards JR, et al. Antimicrobial-resistant pathogens associated with healthcare-associated infections: summary of data reported to the National Healthcare Safety Network at the Centers for Disease Control and Prevention, 2009-2010. Infect Control Hosp Epidemiol 2013;34:1–14.
27. Hidron AI, Edwards JR, Patel J, et al. NHSN annual update: antimicrobial-resistant pathogens associated with healthcare-associated infections: annual summary of data reported to the National Healthcare Safety Network at the Centers for Disease Control and Prevention, 2006-2007. Infect Control Hosp Epidemiol 2008;29:996–1011.
28. Williams REO. Healthy carriage of Staphylococcus aureus: its prevalence and importance. Bacteriol Rev 1963;27:56–71.
29. Huang SS, Platt R. Risk of methicillin-resistant Staphylococcus aureus infection after previous infection or colonization. Clin Infect Dis 2003;36:281–5.
30. Lee AS, de Lencastre H, Garau J, et al. Methicillin-resistant Staphylococcus aureus. Nat Rev Dis Primers 2018;4:1–23.

31. Calfee DP, Salgado CD, Milstone AM, et al. Society for Healthcare Epidemiology of America. Strategies to prevent methicillin-resistant Staphylococcus aureus transmission and infection in acute care hospitals: 2014 update. Infect Control Hosp Epidemiol 2014;35:772–96.
32. Eriksen NH, Espersen F, Rosdahl VT, et al. Carriage of Staphylococcus aureus among 104 healthy persons during a 19-month period. Epidemiol Infect 1995; 115:51–60.
33. Kumar A, Roberts D, Wood KE, et al. Duration of hypotension before initiation of effective antimicrobial therapy is critical determinant of survival in human septic shock. Crit Care Med 2006;34:1589–96.
34. Liu C, Bayer A, Cosgrove SE, et al. Clinical practice guidelines by the Infectious Diseases Society of America for the treatment of methicillin-resistant Staphylococcus aureus infections in adults and children. Clin Infect Dis 2011;52:e18–55.
35. Iversen K, Ihlemann N, Gill SU, et al. Partial oral versus intravenous antibiotic treatment of endocarditis. N Engl J Med 2019;380:415–24.
36. Metlay JP, Waterer GW, Long AC, et al. Diagnosis and treatment of adults with community-acquired pneumonia. An official clinical practice guideline of the American Thoracic Society and Infectious Diseases Society of America. Am J Respir Crit Care Med 2019;200:e45–67.
37. Kalil AC, Metersky ML, Klompas M, et al. Management of adults with hospital-acquired and ventilator-associated pneumonia: 2016 clinical practice guidelines by the Infectious Diseases Society of America and the American Thoracic Society. Clin Infect Dis 2016;63:61–111.
38. Li HK, Rombach I, Zambellas R, et al. Oral versus intravenous antibiotics for bone and joint infection. N Engl J Med 2019;380:425–36.
39. Tunkel AR, Hasbun R, Bhimraj A, et al. 2017 Infectious Diseases Society of America's clinical practice guidelines for healthcare-associated ventriculitis and meningitis. Clin Infect Dis 2017;64:34–65.
40. Hiramatsu K, Hanaki H, Ino T, et al. Methicillin-resistant Staphylococcus aureus clinical strain with reduced vancomycin susceptibility. J Antimicrob Chemother 1997;40:135–6.
41. Weigel LM, Clewell DB, Gill SR, et al. Genetic analysis of a high-level vancomycin-resistant isolate of Staphylococcus aureus. Science 2003;302:1569–71.
42. Sakoulas G, Moise-Broder PA, Schentag J, et al. Relationship of MIC and bactericidal activity to efficacy of vancomycin for treatment of methicillin-resistant Staphylococcus aureus bacteremia. J Clin Microbiol 2004;42:2398–402.
43. Moise PA, Sakoulas G, Forrest A, et al. Vancomycin in vitro bactericidal activity and its relationship to efficacy in clearance of methicillin-resistant Staphylococcus aureus bacteremia. Antimicrob Agents Chemother 2007;57:2582–6.
44. Moise PA, Smyth DS, El-Fawal N, et al. Microbiological effects of prior vancomycin use in patients with methicillin-resistant Staphylococcus aureus bacteraemia. J Antimicrob Chemother 2008;61:85–90.
45. Popovich KJ, Davila S, Chopra V, et al. A tiered approach for preventing methicillin-resistant Staphylococcus aureus infection. Ann Intern Med 2019; 171(7_Supplement):S59–65.

Alcohol and the Hospitalized Patient

Svetlana Chernyavsky, DO, Patricia Dharapak, MD, Jennifer Hui, MD,
Violetta Laskova, MD, Eve Merrill, MD, Kamana Pillay, MD, Evan Siau, MD,
Dahlia Rizk, DO, MPH*

KEYWORDS

- Alcohol use disorder • Hospitalized patients • Cost • Comorbidity • Treatment
- Alcoholic liver disease • Alcohol withdrawal

KEY POINTS

- Alcohol use disorder carries a significant cost burden in the United States and globally.
- Comorbidities associated with excess alcohol use involve multiple organ systems and can often lead to hospitalization.
- Alcohol withdrawal and its appropriate treatment are critical skills required of providers caring for hospitalized patients.
- Alcoholic liver disease and its sequela lead to significant morbidity.
- Treatment options and support for patients exist in helping reduce use of alcohol and its complications.

An estimated 88,000 deaths result from alcohol-related causes annually in the United States, and $249 billion in costs can be attributed to alcohol-related disabilities, work losses, and health care expenditures. Globally, alcohol use is the fifth leading risk factor for premature death and disability.[1]

Alcohol misuse falls into a variety of categories, including binge drinking, which is an ingestion of 5 drinks for men or 4 drinks for women in roughly 2 hours. Legal intoxication in the United States is a blood alcohol concentration greater than 0.08 g/dL. Alcohol use disorder (AUD) as defined by the American Psychiatry Association's *Diagnostic and Statistical Manual of Mental Disorders* (Fifth Edition) (*DSM-V*) integrates 2 *DSM-IV* disorders, alcohol abuse and alcohol dependence, and affects more than 15 million people in the United States alone.[1] It is estimated that more than 20% of admitted patients meet *DSM-V* criteria for AUD and that more than 2 million patients withdraw each year.[2,3]

Department of Medicine, Mt Sinai Beth Israel, Icahn School of Medicine, 16th Street and 1st Avenue, New York, NY 10010, USA
* Corresponding author.
E-mail address: Dahlia.Rizk@mountsinai.org

Med Clin N Am 104 (2020) 681–694
https://doi.org/10.1016/j.mcna.2020.02.007
0025-7125/20/© 2020 Elsevier Inc. All rights reserved.

Patients with AUD can suffer from a myriad of complications affecting essentially every organ system. The risk of cirrhosis, gastrointestinal hemorrhage, upper airway and gastrointestinal cancers, dementia, and malnutrition is sharply increased in those with frequent alcohol use. Consuming 3 or more drinks daily has been linked to hypertension, and heavy drinkers are at increased risk for coronary artery disease, arrhythmias, and heart failure.[4] The hospitalized alcohol-dependent patient also has a higher prevalence of polysubstance abuse and mental health comorbidities.[5]

NEUROLOGIC MANIFESTATIONS

Alcohol acts as a central nervous system depressant similar to benzodiazepines or barbiturates. The neurologic manifestations of alcohol withdrawal syndrome (AWS) occur when this central nervous system depressant is removed and include alcoholic hallucinosis, delirium tremens (DT), withdrawal seizures, and Wernicke encephalopathy (WE). Considering the rapid rate of alcohol clearance in patients with chronic alcohol use, the clinical manifestations of withdrawal begin as early as 2 hours from the last drink and typically occur within the first 6 to 8 hours (**Fig. 1**). Minor withdrawal symptoms, such as diaphoresis and headache, typically occur in this timeframe. A subset of patients with AWS or AUD will develop late-onset or chronic neurologic manifestations, which include Korsakoff syndrome (KS), alcohol-induced psychotic disorders (AIPS), or late-onset seizures.

Alcohol hallucinosis characterized by auditory hallucinations during or after a period of heavy drinking occurs in about 1% of patients with AUD. About 80% to 90% of patients report hallucinations exclusively during alcohol withdrawal, although hallucinations may also occur while consuming alcohol. It is an acute disorder with a typical onset 12 to 24 hours from the last drink and usually resolves in less than a week when treated.[6]

DT is diagnosed if a patient meets the criteria for both alcohol withdrawal and delirium.[7] DT may or may not include hallucinations and is distinguished from alcoholic hallucinosis by the presence of autonomic hyperactivity, including tachycardia,

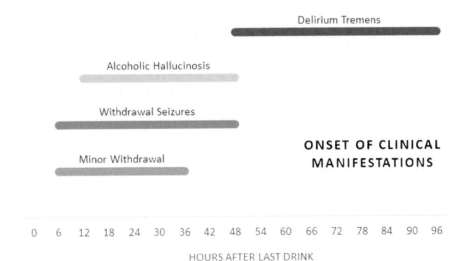

Fig. 1. Onset of clinical manifestations in alcohol withdrawal syndrome. (*Data from* Refs.[2,6,8,10])

hypertension, fever, and diaphoresis. DT occurs in about 3% to 5% of alcohol withdrawal cases with a typical onset 2 to 4 days from the last drink, and lasts 2 to 3 days, although durations of up to 8 days have been reported.[8] Fortunately, the mortality has historically declined from 15% to 35% to 1% to 5%.[9]

Withdrawal seizures occur in 10% to 30% of alcohol withdrawal cases, with the onset of seizure usually 6 to 48 hours from the last drink.[10] Alcohol affects the neurotransmitter receptors, including gamma-aminobutyric acid (GABA) and N-methyl-D-aspartate (NMDA) receptors, and its abrupt cessation can trigger activation of neuronal networks in the brainstem, which may be the underlying mechanism that contributes to withdrawal seizures.[11] The presenting seizure is typically a generalized tonic-clonic seizure, although partial-onset seizures likely occur more frequently than previously recognized. Although the escalation of a withdrawal seizure into status epilepticus is rare, AUD is a major precipitant of 9% to 25% of status epilepticus cases.[12]

WE and KS are neurologic disorders resulting from 2 separate stages of thiamine deficiency. WE is an acute manifestation, whereas KS is a late neuropsychiatric syndrome caused by untreated WE. Classically, WE is a clinical diagnosis with triad of encephalopathy, oculomotor abnormalities (nystagmus, lateral gaze palsy), and in 10% of the cases, gait ataxia and cerebellar dysfunction.[13] Coma, hypotension, hypothermia, and vestibular dysfunction may also be present with WE. About 80% of patients with untreated WE progress to the largely irreversible KS, characterized by marked episodic memory impairment that is out of proportion to other cognitive functions. Additional cognitive and behavioral dysfunction, such as executive dysfunction, flattened affect, apathy, and lack of insight, may also be present.[14]

The diagnosis of alcohol-induced psychotic syndrome (AIPS) should be suspected when psychotic symptoms are prominent and exceeds the perceptual disturbance normally seen in alcohol intoxication or withdrawal, or consciousness disturbance seen in delirium. The lifetime prevalence of AIPS is 0.5%. AIPS and DT are assumed to be different manifestations of the same process, although the prognosis of AIPS is better than DT.[15]

In addition to acute withdrawal seizure, patients with AUD may also develop seizures that occur remotely from alcohol consumption. The hypothesized causes include direct alcohol toxicity to the brain, concurrent prior undiagnosed brain injuries, anoxic encephalopathy from prior status epilepticus, or repeated cycles of alcohol exposure and withdrawal through a process known as kindling.[12] AUD and AWS have also been associated with acute/chronic myopathy, peripheral neuropathy, cognitive impairment, ventricular enlargement, and cerebellar degeneration.[16]

LIVER DISEASE

Patients with excess alcohol intake are susceptible to developing alcoholic liver disease (ALD), including alcoholic steatosis, alcoholic hepatitis (AH), and alcoholic cirrhosis (AC). Individuals are at risk with consumption of greater than 30 g per day or about 2 standard drinks (at ~14 g each, equivalent to 12 oz. beer, 8 oz. malt liquor, 5 oz. wine, or 1.5 oz. distilled spirits). Women have greater susceptibility to liver injury than men for a given quantity of alcohol, and 1 standard drink per day is recommended as a safe limit.[17] However, liver toxicity is not dictated by the quantity ingested alone, and only a small percentage (<20%) of patients will progress to advanced liver disease despite heavy intake (>100 g/d). Genetic factors, obesity, tobacco use, comorbid liver disease, such as chronic hepatitis B virus (HBV) or hepatitis C virus (HCV) infection, nonalcoholic fatty liver disease, and hemochromatosis are associated with an elevated risk for hepatic damage with concomitant alcohol intake.[18]

Virtually all individuals with significant alcohol intake (>40 g/d) develop alcoholic fatty liver, which is typically asymptomatic.[19] The diagnosis is made in the setting of known heavy alcohol use along with compatible imaging and/or laboratory findings (mild transaminitis with aspartate aminotransferase [AST] > alanine aminotransferase [ALT], serum bilirubin less than 3 mg/dL, elevated gamma-glutamyl transferase levels). Alcohol-induced steatosis alone is usually benign and regresses after several weeks of abstinence.[20]

Less than one-third of patients with steatosis and ongoing alcohol use evolve to alcoholic steatohepatitis (ASH), diagnosed histologically by characteristic hepatocyte injury, inflammation, or fibrosis. ASH may be clinically silent or manifest as overt AH, a clinical syndrome comprising progressive jaundice (within 8 weeks), right upper quadrant pain, fever, and constitutional symptoms. A probable clinical diagnosis of AH may be made in the setting of heavy alcohol use greater than 5 years with active use within 4 weeks, sudden onset of jaundice with bilirubin greater than 3 mg/dL, AST:ALT greater than 1.5, and AST greater than 50 but less than 400 IU/L in the absence of other causes.[21] A commonly used scoring system for assessing AH severity is Maddrey discriminant function (DMF), which accounts for prothrombin time and bilirubin. AH cases with DMF $\geq$32 are severe, with an estimated mortality greater than 30% at 28 days.[22] The model for end-stage liver disease (MELD) score, which uses international normalized ratio and incorporates renal function, is also validated for predicting short-term mortality at 30 and 90 days in AH, with scores $\geq$21 signifying severe disease.[23] Treatment of all AH involves alcohol abstinence, nutritional support, comprehensive screening and treatment of any concurrent infection, and renal protective measures, such as avoiding dehydration.

For severe AH, the American College of Gastroenterology 2018 guidelines recommend hospitalization and treatment with corticosteroids if there are no absolute contraindications, such as active HBV, HCV, and *Mycobacterium tuberculosis* infections. Other infections, uncontrolled diabetes, or gastrointestinal bleeding are relative contraindications.[24] Prednisolone is typically prescribed at 40 mg daily for 28 days, with or without a subsequent taper. The efficacy of corticosteroids is still a matter of debate. STOPAH, the largest randomized controlled trial studying the effect of prednisolone and pentoxifylline in severe AH, found a statistically nonsignificant reduction in mortality at 28 days (14% vs 17%) but no improvement in death or liver transplantation rates at 90 days and 1 year.[25] Moreover, a 2019 Cochrane Review found very low certainty of evidence on mortality, health-related quality of life, and harm and could not conclude on the benefit of steroids.[26] Pentoxifylline use in severe AH may potentially reduce the incidence of hepatorenal syndrome, but has not been shown to have a survival benefit compared with placebo, in combination with prednisolone, or as salvage for steroid nonresponse and is therefore not recommended for routine use.[27,28] N-acetylcysteine, an antioxidant, shows promise as an adjunct to prednisolone for treatment of severe AH, with a significant decrease in mortality at 1 month compared with prednisolone alone (8% vs 24%) in one randomized control trial, although additional research is needed.[29]

About 8% to 20% of patients with ASH progress to AC, which is suggested by signs and symptoms of portal hypertension, imaging findings of hepatic nodularity, or elastography.[24] Prognosis may be assessed with MELD and Child-Pugh scores, but mortalities for this population are high even without decompensation (ascites, bleeding, or encephalopathy) at initial diagnosis. In one Danish study, AC patients without any of the above complications at diagnosis had 17% mortality at 1 year and 57% at 5 years, a majority from direct complications of ALD, as well as hepatocellular and other cancers.[30]

Treatment of AUD is paramount, because persistent alcohol consumption (>10 g/d) has been identified as the strongest modifiable risk factor impacting mortality in AC.[31] In addition, patients with decompensated AC, Child-Pugh C, or MELD-Na $\geq$ 21 should be referred for liver transplantation after screening for comorbid medical conditions and psychosocial assessment. Most programs require 6 months of abstinence before transplant listing.[18] Early transplant referral may be considered for select patients presenting with a first episode of severe AH refractory to medical treatment, because most will not survive to 6 months.[32]

HEMATOLOGICAL EFFECTS

Alcohol has both direct and indirect toxic effects on all cell lines, mediated by metabolites, which inhibit hematopoiesis. It causes structural changes to blood cells and results in fewer precursor cells as well as cell dysfunction.[33–36] Indirectly, alcohol contributes to each cytopenia through alcohol-induced dysfunction of multiple organ systems. AC can cause thrombocytopenia as well as decreased red blood cell production. Alcohol-induced portal hypertension causes hypersplenism and can result in one or more cytopenias through sequestration. Heavy alcohol use can also lead to ulcers with resultant gastrointestinal blood loss.[33,34] Fortunately, the direct toxic effects of alcohol on the bone marrow can reverse within a few weeks of abstinence.

Alcohol can lead to a variety of anemias, including sideroblastic, megaloblastic, hemolytic, and iron deficiency. Acting directly on the bone marrow, it produces large vacuoles in the precursor red blood cells secondary to alcohol-induced cell membrane damage, which can also predispose red blood cells to hemolysis. In addition, gastrointestinal absorption of folate and iron is inhibited, also leading to anemia.[36]

White blood cell maturation, production, and neutrophil function are affected. Neutrophil delivery to areas of infection is inhibited, and alcohol reduces neutrophil adherence to blood vessel walls causing decreased neutrophil responsiveness to leukotriene signaling. Alcohol is also thought to inhibit macrophage and monocyte function, but not their quantity.[36]

Platelet count and function (including aggregation) are likewise affected. Similar to red blood cells, platelet precursors (megakaryocytes) are prone to vacuolization, which may alter the function and lifespan of platelets.[36] Coagulopathies related to thrombocytopenias and fibrinogen production also contribute to acute blood loss anemia.[35]

MALNUTRITION AND ELECTROLYTE DERANGEMENTS

Alcohol has considerable energy value (7.1 kcal/g) but provides "empty calories," because it contains few micronutrients, vitamins, and minerals. Malnutrition is present in 20% to 90% of heavy alcohol consumers with ALD, and sarcopenia (muscle loss) can reach levels of nearly 70%.[37] For those with ALD, mortality risk increases in direct proportion to the extent of malnutrition, approaching 80% in those with severe malnutrition.[38]

Primary malnutrition is caused by displacement of other dietary elements with alcoholic intake.[39] Secondary malnutrition results from maldigestion or malabsorption of nutrients, primarily thiamine, folate, and zinc. Typically, these are the consequence of alcohol-induced gastrointestinal complications, such as pancreatic insufficiency and intestinal lactase deficiency.[39] In turn, the presence of nutritional deficiencies further potentiates ethanol hepatotoxicity.

Alcohol use is the most important risk factor for thiamine deficiency as alcohol intake decreases thiamine absorption in the small intestine. The prevalence of WE among patients with alcoholism varies from 12.5% to 35% compared with 1.5% in the general population.[40] Some WE patients supplemented with thiamine alone will have partial or no clinical improvement. Although it is unclear what actual dose is truly effective, treating WE traditionally entails intravenous or intramuscular doses of thiamine, then continuing oral thiamine while hospitalized or while still drinking.[41] Adding supplemental magnesium may lead to an improvement in cognition and increased thiamine absorption.[42]

Zinc deficiency is frequently observed in heavy alcohol drinkers and has a wide range of manifestations, including skin lesions, impaired wound healing, poor liver regeneration, altered mental status, and altered immunity. Fifty milligrams of elemental zinc taken with meals daily is recommended for treatment in patients with ALD.[43]

Electrolyte depletion, notably hypomagnesemia, hypokalemia, hypophosphatemia, and hypocalcemia, is also very common in this setting. Hypomagnesemia is often due to low magnesium intake, diarrheal losses, and respiratory alkalosis. Hypokalemia typically results from hypomagnesemia, compounded by alcohol's diuretic properties, which cause increased urinary potassium excretion, and poor dietary intake.[44] Excess phosphorus excretion, hypomagnesemia, metabolic acidosis, and respiratory alkalosis contribute to hypophosphatemia.[45] As such, it is important to evaluate and aggressively replete electrolyte deficiencies to prevent cardiac, respiratory, and neurologic complications. A suggested initial therapy in patients with multiple electrolyte deficiencies is a solution of 1 L of 5% dextrose in 0.45% saline with 20 mmol of potassium phosphate and 4 mL of 50% magnesium sulfate.[46]

TREATMENT OF ALCOHOL WITHDRAWAL

Benzodiazepines are the mainstay of alcohol withdrawal treatment and prevention. They work by stimulating the GABA receptor, resulting in a reduction of neuronal activity. The reduction in neuronal activity leads to a sedative effect and slows the progression of withdrawal symptoms.[47] The most studied benzodiazepines for the treatment and prevention of alcohol withdrawal are chlordiazepoxide, diazepam, lorazepam, and oxazepam.[47–52] Although no specific benzodiazepine is recommended for AWS, long-acting benzodiazepines with active metabolites (chlordiazepoxide, diazepam) are preferred for patients with minimal comorbidities.[53] Lorazepam appears to be the safest choice when treating elderly patients and those with liver disease.[54] Shorter-acting benzodiazepines should be considered in patients with severe lung disease or those prone to respiratory depression.

The preferred route of administration of benzodiazepines should be based on the severity of withdrawal. Intravenous administration has a rapid onset and is the route of choice in patients with seizure activity or DTs. In cases of benzodiazepine overdose, flumazenil injection may be indicated and used.[55] Once a patient has clinically responded to intravenous administration of a benzodiazepine, oral formulations are commonly used (**Table 1**).

In mild withdrawal or in the outpatient setting, oral administration is favored. For some patients, nonpharmacologic interventions are the first-line approach and may be the only management required. Nonpharmacologic measures include frequent reassurance, reality orientation, and nursing care.[57] A quiet room without dark shadows, noises, and other excessive stimuli is recommended.[58]

Multiple strategies are available for the administration of benzodiazepines once withdrawal is diagnosed. Symptom-triggered therapy (STT) is one approach. The Clinical Institute Withdrawal Assessment–Alcohol Revised (CIWA-Ar) scale for alcohol assessment is a validated tool that has been commonly used in clinical trials to

Table 1
Comparison of commonly used benzodiazepines for alcohol withdrawal syndrome

	Chlordiazepoxide	Diazepam	Lorazepam	Oxazepam
Route of administration	po	po, IV, rectal	po, IV, IM	po
Dose equivalence, mg	25	5	1	15
Speed of onset	Intermediate	Rapid	Intermediate	Slow
Active metabolites	Yes (hepatically metabolized)	Yes (hepatically metabolized)	No	No
Half-life	Long	Long	Short	Short
Lipid solubility	Less lipophilic than diazepam; slower onset of action	Highly lipophilic with rapid onset of action	Less lipophilic than diazepam; slower onset of action	Less lipophilic than diazepam; slower onset of action
Effect of renal disease	No dose adjustment[a]	No dose adjustment	Half-life increased; elimination impaired	No dose adjustment

[a] No dose adjustment is required by the manufacturer, but per current recommendations, the dose should be reduced by 50% for those with renal impairment (CrCl <10 mL/min).[56]
   Data from Refs.[53,56,60,61]

quantify and monitor alcohol withdrawal severity and benzodiazepine titration treatment of patients with mild to moderate withdrawal.[48–52,59,60] The CIWA-Ar is quick and takes into account 10 common signs and symptoms, with scoring based on provider observations and patient reporting.[59,60] The use of CIWA-Ar has several limitations, including diversity of protocols and patients in studies examining its use and the need for appropriately educated staff to perform the assessment. Current evidence supports STT in most patients because it can reduce benzodiazepine use, reduce adverse events related to benzodiazepine use, and decrease length of stay.[47–52] Fixed dose regimens are another option for the treatment of alcohol withdrawal, especially for patients who are unable to convey symptoms. A fixed dose regimen is preferred when the intense monitoring required for STT is unable to be performed.[61]

A symptom-monitored loading (SML) dose is another means to treat alcohol withdrawal, especially for patients with a history of severe alcohol withdrawal syndrome (SAWS). With SML, a single loading dose of benzodiazepine is given immediately on presentation, and then the patient is monitored for signs of withdrawal (ie, using CIWA-Ar). This strategy allows the use and advantages of the STT, while taking into account the patient's past medical history and acute medical illness.[61–63]

Rapid loading with close monitoring is another titration method but is recommended only in patients with DT. This method usually involves intravenous benzodiazepine administration at frequent intervals with close monitoring.[61,62] The Prediction of Alcohol Withdrawal Severity Score (PAWSS) is a 10-point questionnaire and was the first validated tool for the prediction of SAWS in medically ill, hospitalized individuals. Wood and colleagues[64] demonstrated that a history of DTs with a baseline systolic blood pressure of 140 mm Hg or higher on admission was associated with increased risk of SAWS. Given the association of SAWS with a PAWSS of 4 or more, prophylaxis and/or treatment may be indicated to help shorten hospitalization and decrease associated care costs.

Patients with acute trauma, DTs, or persistent withdrawal seizures are typically admitted to the intensive care unit (ICU), but others remain at risk for deterioration.[60,65] There is no universal guideline for ICU evaluation. Carlson and colleagues[65] suggests criteria for ICU admission to include those in alcohol withdrawal with cardiac disease, hemodynamic instability, severe electrolyte abnormalities, marked acid-base disturbances, respiratory abnormalities, serious infections, history of SAWS, and the need for frequent high doses of sedatives.[65]

OTHER AGENTS

An alternative to conventional benzodiazepine treatment is phenobarbital, a long-acting barbiturate. Phenobarbital has similar pharmacokinetics to the benzodiazepines, including simultaneous effects on GABA and NMDA receptors, and has been proposed as a treatment option for DTs. Current research offers only modest guidance as to the safety and efficacy of phenobarbital in managing AWS in hospitalized patients. Nelson and colleagues[66] found that incorporating phenobarbital into a benzodiazepine-based protocol or as sole agent led to similar rates of ICU admission, length of stay, and need for mechanical ventilation in patients treated for alcohol withdrawal in the emergency department. Adverse effects with phenobarbital, including dizziness and drowsiness, rarely occurred.[67] Further studies are needed to determine dosing and to further characterize appropriate use.

Gabapentin is a promising treatment option in AWS and may reduce the need for benzodiazepines. Gabapentin works by exerting GABA-mimetic properties, thus mitigating the physiologic imbalance that contributes to AWS. Common side effects include dizziness, drowsiness, ataxia, diarrhea, nausea, and vomiting. Although misuse is associated with current or past opioid, cocaine, and benzodiazepine abuse, AUD does not appear to be a predictor for gabapentin misuse.[68,69]

In several small studies, gabapentin monotherapy was found to be comparable to benzodiazepines in the treatment of mild to moderate AWS, and to be efficacious in reducing cravings, improving mood, improving anxiety, and improving sleep with less sedation.[70,71] Gabapentin appears more effective at lowering CIWA-Ar scores and superior in preventing relapse with no difference in length of hospital stay when compared with benzodiazepines.[70,72,73] However, given the small sample sizes of these studies, differing methods, and study participants, the generalizability of these results is limited.

Alternative agents, such as antipsychotics (eg, haloperidol), centrally acting alpha-2 agonists (eg, clonidine), beta-blockers, and baclofen (selective GABA-B receptor agonist), may attenuate the symptoms of withdrawal but are not routinely recommended because of limited evidence for their efficacy and known potential for harm (including masking symptoms of progressive withdrawal and lowering seizure threshold). Several anticonvulsants (valproic acid, levetiracetam, topiramate, and zonisamide) also showed limited efficacy in reducing withdrawal symptoms but lack support for routine use as monotherapy to prevent withdrawal seizures or DT.[74]

NONPHARMACOLOGIC INTERVENTIONS

AUD is a complex and chronic, relapsing syndrome that often requires multiple treatment targets. Although the short-term remission rate for those who receive treatment is 20% to 50%, the estimated long-term relapse rate is still 20% to 80%.[75]

Psychosocial interventions can be effective, and all should be encouraged to participate. Brief interventions may suffice for those with mild disorders as defined by *DSM-V*. For moderate to severe AUD, several evidence-supported therapies are available (**Table 2**), each of comparable effectiveness.[76,77] The response to treatment and the intervention selected will vary with the individual.[76,78] There is mixed evidence on whether combining medication and psychosocial interventions leads to better outcomes than with either method alone.[79]

There is outcome benefit in matching AUD severity and level of cognitive function to the treatment setting. In particular, patients with high alcohol problem severity and/or low cognitive function benefit most from inpatient treatment.[80] The American Society of Addiction Medicine offers an approach to identify the appropriate level of care based on the severity of substance use disorder. With levels of severity ranging from 0.5 to 4.0, level 4 patients are recommended for medically managed intensive inpatient services, whereas those at level 0.5 are recommended for early intervention.[81] Local availability and insurance coverage of inpatient and outpatient treatment programs will vary.

Concurrent drug use and mental health issues are common among people with AUD and associated with poorer AUD treatment outcomes. Routine screening for both is recommended when treating AUD, and the coexisting disorder should be treated according to practice guidelines. Food and housing insecurities are potential stressors that can adversely impact treatment outcomes. Partnering with social services to identify and mitigate competing socioeconomic stressors can improve the likelihood of treatment success.

DRUGS FOR ALCOHOL ABSTINENCE

There are several medication options to reduce the risk of relapse after successful alcohol detoxification. The first drug approved for this indication was disulfiram, an aversive agent that causes dysphoria, nausea, and vomiting when used with alcohol. There have been mixed reports on its effectiveness, mainly because of poor compliance.[82] Naltrexone can be used to block the euphoric feeling associated with alcohol use and has been shown to increase the time to next relapse and decrease cravings

Table 2 Evidence based nonpharmacologic interventions	
Brief interventions	For example, simple expressions of concern expressed by a clinician
Cognitive behavioral therapy	Individuals learn how their thought processes contribute to behaviors and work on developing adaptive ways of behaving
Motivational enhancement or Interviewing therapy	Individuals explore and resolve attitudes and ambivalence about change
Mutual-help groups	For example, 12-step support groups Helps individuals work toward abstinence through group sharing and support
Contingency management	Incentives are offered to discourage substance use/encourage abstinence

Adapted from Campbell EJ, Lawrence AJ, Perry CJ. New steps for treating alcohol use disorder. Psychopharmacology (Berl) 2018;235(6):1759-1773; and Martin GW, Rehm J. The Effectiveness of Psychosocial Modalities in the Treatment of Alcohol Problems in Adults: A Review of the Evidence. Can J Psychiatry 2012;57(6):350-358; with permission.

after 12 weeks. However, naltrexone can precipitate withdrawal in those using opiates and is contraindicated in that population.[83] Acamprosate can help reduce chronic withdrawal symptoms and maintain abstinence for weeks to months as demonstrated by several meta-analyses.[84] In patients with AC without hepatic encephalopathy, baclofen (titrated to 10 mg 3 times daily) appears efficacious in lengthening the duration of abstinence without significant adverse events.[85] Last, gabapentin has also shown promise in maintenance of abstinence.[86]

DISCLOSURE

The authors have nothing to disclose.

REFERENCES

1. CDC– fact sheets: "alcohol use and health–alcohol". Atlanta, GA: Centers for Disease Control and Prevention; 2018.
2. Rawlani V, et al. Treatment of the hospitalized alcohol-dependent patient with alcohol withdrawal syndrome. Internet J Intern Med 2008;8(1).
3. Grant BF, Goldstein RB, Saha TD, et al. Epidemiology of DSM-5 alcohol use disorder: results from the National Epidemiologic Survey on Alcohol and Related Conditions III. JAMA Psychiatry 2015;72:757–66.
4. Greenspon AJ, Schaal SF. The "holiday heart": electrophysiologic studies of alcohol effects in alcoholics. Ann Intern Med 1983;98(2):135–9.
5. Castillo-Carniglia A, Keyes K, Hasin D, et al. Psychiatric comorbidities in alcohol use disorder. Lancet Psychiatry 2019;6(12):1068–80.
6. Narasimha VL, Patley R, Shukla L, et al. Phenomenology and course of alcoholic hallucinosis. J Dual Diagn 2019;15(3):172–6.
7. Association AP. Diagnostic and statistical manual of mental disorders (DSM-5®). Washington, DC: American Psychiatric Pub; 2013.
8. Schuckit MA. Recognition and management of withdrawal delirium (delirium tremens). N Engl J Med 2014;371(22):2109–13.
9. Hasin DS, Stinson FS, Ogburn E, et al. Prevalence, correlates, disability, and comorbidity of DSM-IV alcohol abuse and dependence in the United States: results from the National Epidemiologic Survey on Alcohol and Related Conditions. Arch Gen Psychiatry 2007;64(7):830–42.
10. Victor M, Brausch C. The role of abstinence in the genesis of alcoholic epilepsy. Epilepsia 2007;8(1):1–20.
11. Rogawski MA. Update on the neurobiology of alcohol withdrawal seizures. Epilepsy Curr 2005;5(6):225–30.
12. Hillbom M, Pieninkeroinen I, Leone M. Seizures in alcohol-dependent patients: epidemiology, pathophysiology and management. CNS Drugs 2003;17(14): 1013–30.
13. Sinha S, Kataria A, Kolla BP, et al. Wernicke encephalopathy-clinical pearls. Mayo Clin Proc 2019;94(6):1065–72.
14. Arts NJ, Walvoort SJ, Kessels RP. Korsakoff's syndrome: a critical review. Neuropsychiatr Dis Treat 2017;13:2875–90.
15. Perala J, Kuoppasalmi K, Pirkola S, et al. Alcohol-induced psychotic disorder and delirium in the general population. Br J Psychiatry 2010;197(3):200–6.
16. Shield KD, Parry C, Rehm J. Chronic diseases and conditions related to alcohol use. Alcohol Res 2013;35(2):155–73.

17. Dietary Guidelines for Americans 2015-2020. Office of Disease Prevention and Health Promotion Website. Available at: http://health.gov/dietaryguidelines/2015/guidelines/appendix-9/. Accessed October 10, 2019.

18. Crabb DW, Im GY, Szabo G, et al. Diagnosis and treatment of alcohol-related liver diseases: 2019 practice guidance from the American Association for the Study of Liver Diseases. Hepatology 2019. https://doi.org/10.1002/hep.30866.

19. Seitz HK, Bataller R, Cortez-Pinto H, et al. Alcoholic liver disease. Nat Rev Dis Primers 2018;4(1):16.

20. Tang-Barton P, Vas W, Weissman J, et al. Focal fatty liver lesions in alcoholic liver disease: a broadened spectrum of CT appearances. Gastrointest Radiol 1985; 10:133.

21. Crabb DW, Bataller R, Chalasani NP, et al. Standard definitions and common data elements for clinical trials in patients with alcoholic hepatitis: recommendation from the NIAAA Alcoholic Hepatitis Consortia. Gastroenterology 2016;150: 785–90.

22. Gholam PM. Prognosis and prognostic scoring models for alcoholic liver disease and acute alcoholic hepatitis. Clin Liver Dis 2016;20:491–7.

23. Dunn W, Jamil LH, Brown LS, et al. MELD accurately predicts mortality in patients with alcoholic hepatitis. Hepatology 2005;41(2):353–8.

24. Singal AK, Bataller R, Ahn J, et al. ACG clinical guideline: alcoholic liver disease. Am J Gastroenterol 2018;113:175–94.

25. Thursz MR, Richardson P, Allison M, et al. Prednisolone or pentoxifylline for alcoholic hepatitis. N Engl J Med 2015;372:1619–28.

26. Pavlov CS, Varganova DL, Casazza G, et al. Glucocorticosteroids for people with alcoholic hepatitis. Cochrane Database Syst Rev 2019;(4):CD001511.

27. Akriviadis E, Botla R, Briggs W, et al. Pentoxifylline improves short-term survival in severe acute alcoholic hepatitis: a double-blind, placebo-controlled trial. Gastroenterology 2000;119:1637–48.

28. Parker R, Armstrong MJ, Corbett C, et al. Systematic review: pentoxifylline for the treatment of severe alcoholic hepatitis. Aliment Pharmacol Ther 2013;37:845–54.

29. Nguyen-Khac E, Thevenot T, Piquet MA, et al. Glucocorticoids plus N-acetylcysteine in severe alcoholic hepatitis. N Engl J Med 2011;365:1781–9.

30. Jepsen P, Ott P, Andersen PK, et al. Clinical course of alcoholic liver cirrhosis: a Danish population-based cohort study. Hepatology 2010;51:1675–82.

31. Bell H, Jahnsen J, Kittang E, et al. Long-term prognosis of patients with alcoholic liver cirrhosis: a 15-year follow-up study of 100 Norwegian patients admitted to one unit. Scand J Gastroenterol 2004;39:858–63.

32. Mathurin P, Moreno C, Samuel D, et al. Early liver transplantation for severe alcoholic hepatitis. N Engl J Med 2011;365:1790–800.

33. Girard DE, Kumar KL, McAfee JH. Hematologic effects of acute and chronic alcohol abuse. Hematol Oncol Clin North Am 1987;1(2):321–34.

34. Latvala J, Parkkila S, Niemelä O. Excess alcohol consumption is common in patients with cytopenia: studies in blood and bone marrow cells. Alcohol Clin Exp Res 2004;28:619–24.

35. Elanchezhian, Yoganandh T, Mayilsamy S, et al. Comparison of hematological parameters between alcoholics and non-alcoholics. Int J Res Med Sci 2017;5: 5041–7.

36. Ballard HS. The hematological complications of alcoholism. Alcohol Health Res World 1997;21(1):42–52.

37. Dasarathy S. Nutrition and alcoholic liver disease: effects of alcoholism on nutrition, effects of nutrition on alcoholic liver disease, and nutritional therapies for alcoholic liver disease (review). Clin Liver Dis 2016;20(3):535–50.
38. O'Shear R. Alcoholic liver disease. Hepatology 2010;51(1):307–28.
39. Lieber C. Alcohol: its metabolism and interaction with nutrients. Annu Rev Nutr 2000;20:295–430.
40. Polegato BF, Pereira AG, Azevedo PS, et al. Role of thiamine in health and disease. Nutr Clin Pract 2019;34(4):558–64.
41. Day E, Bentham P, Callaghan R, et al. Thiamine for Wernicke-Korsakoff syndrome in people at risk from alcohol abuse. Cochrane Database Syst Rev 2004;(1):CD004033.
42. Jeynes K, Gibson EL. The importance of nutrition in aiding recovery from substance use disorders: a review. Drug Alcohol Depend 2017;179:229–39.
43. Barve S, Chen SY, Kirpich I, et al. Development, prevention, and treatment of alcohol-induced organ injury: the role of nutrition. Alcohol Res 2017;38(2):e1–14.
44. Elisaf M, Merkouropoulos M, Tsianos EV, et al. Acid-base and electrolyte abnormalities in alcoholic patients. Miner Electrolyte Metab 1994;20(5):274–81.
45. Elisaf MS, Siamopoulos KC. Mechanisms of hypophosphataemia in alcoholic patients. Int J Clin Pract 1997;51(8):501–3.
46. Palmer B, Clegg DJ. Electrolyte disturbances in patients with chronic alcohol-use disorder. N Engl J Med 2017;377(14):1368–77.
47. Amato L, Minozzi S, Vecchi S, et al. Benzodiazepines for alcohol withdrawal. Cochrane Database Syst Rev 2010;(3):CD005063.
48. Saitz R, Mayo-Smith MF, Roberts MS, et al. Individualized treatment for alcohol withdrawal. A randomized double-blind controlled trial. JAMA 1994;272(7):519–23.
49. Jaeger TM, Lohr RH, Pankratz VS. Symptom-triggered therapy for alcohol withdrawal syndrome in medical inpatients. Mayo Clin Proc 2001;76:695–701.
50. Daeppen JB, Gache P, Landry U, et al. Symptom-triggered vs fixed-schedule doses of benzodiazepine for alcohol withdrawal: a randomized treatment trial. Arch Intern Med 2002;162:1117–21.
51. Weaver MF, Hoffman HJ, Johnson RE, et al. Alcohol withdrawal pharmacotherapy for inpatients with medical comorbidity. J Addict Dis 2006;25:17–24.
52. Reoux JP, Miller K. Routine hospital alcohol detoxification practice compared to symptom triggered management with an objective withdrawal scale (CIWA-Ar). Am J Addict 2000;9:135–44.
53. Bird RD, Makela EH. Alcohol withdrawal: what is the benzodiazepine of choice? Ann Pharmacother 1994;28:67.
54. Peppers MP. Benzodiazepines for alcohol withdrawal in the elderly and in patients with liver disease. Pharmacotherapy 1996;16:49–57.
55. An H, Godwin J. Flumazenil in benzodiazepine overdose. CMAJ 2016;188(17–18):E537.
56. Kim PM, Weinstein SL. Benzodiazepines. Johns Hopkins Psychiatry Guide; 2016.
57. Naranjo CA, Sellers EM, Chater K, et al. Nonpharmacologic intervention in acute alcohol withdrawal. Clin Pharmacol Ther 1983;34:214–9.
58. Blondell RD. Ambulatory detoxification of patients with alcohol dependence. Am Fam Physician 2005;71:495–502.
59. Sullivan JT, Sykora K, Schneiderman J, et al. Assessment of alcohol withdrawal: the revised Clinical Institute Withdrawal Assessment for Alcohol scale (CIWA-Ar). Br J Addict 1989;84(11):1353–7.

60. Gortney JS, Raub JN, Patel P, et al. Alcohol withdrawal syndrome in medical patients. Cleve Clin J Med 2016;83:67–79.

61. Kattimani S, Bharadwaj B. Clinical management of alcohol withdrawal: a systematic review. Ind Psychiatry J 2013;22(2):100–8.

62. Saitz R, O'Malley SS. Pharmacotherapies for alcohol abuse. Withdrawal and treatment. Med Clin North Am 1997;81:881–907.

63. Devenyi P, Harrison ML. Prevention of alcohol withdrawal seizures with oral diazepam loading. Can Med Assoc J 1985;132:798–800.

64. Wood E, Albarqouni L, Tkachuk S, et al. Will This Hospitalized Patient Develop Severe Alcohol Withdrawal Syndrome?: The Rational Clinical Examination Systematic Review. JAMA 2018;320:825.

65. Carlson RW, Keske B, Cortez D. Alcohol withdrawal syndrome: alleviating symptoms, preventing progression. J Crit Illn 1998;13:311.

66. Nelson AC, Kehoe J, Sankoff J, et al. Benzodiazepines vs barbiturates for alcohol withdrawal: analysis of 3 different treatment protocols. Am J Emerg Med 2019; 37(4):733–6.

67. Hammond DA, Rowe JM, Wong A, et al. Patient outcomes associated with phenobarbital use with or without benzodiazepines for alcohol withdrawal syndrome: a systematic review. Hosp Pharm 2017;52(9):607–16.

68. Bockbrader HN, Wesche D, Miller R, et al. A comparison of the pharmacokinetics and pharmacodynamics of pregabalin and gabapentin. Clin Pharmacokinet 2010;49:661–9.

69. Evoy KE, Morrison MD, Saklad SR. Abuse and misuse of pregabalin and gabapentin. Drugs 2017;77:403–26.

70. Leung JG, Hall-Flavin D, Nelson S, et al. The role of gabapentin in the management of alcohol withdrawal and dependence. Ann Pharmacother 2015;49(8): 897–906.

71. Leung JG, Rakocevic DG, Allen ND, et al. Use of a gabapentin protocol for the management of alcohol withdrawal: a preliminary experience expanding from the consultation-liaison psychiatry service. Psychosomatics 2018;59(5):496–505.

72. Myrick H, Malcolm R, Randall PK, et al. A double blind trial of gabapentin versus lorazepam in the treatment of alcohol withdrawal. Alcohol Clin Exp Res 2009;33: 1582–8.

73. Bonnet U, Hamzavi-Abedi R, Specka M, et al. An open trial of gabapentin in acute alcohol withdrawal using an oral loading protocol. Alcohol Alcohol 2010; 45(2):143–5.

74. Hammond CJ, Niciu MJ, Drew S, et al. Anticonvulsants for the treatment of alcohol withdrawal syndrome and alcohol use disorders. CNS Drugs 2015; 29(4):293–311.

75. Moos RH, Moos BS. Rates and predictors of relapse after natural and treated remission from alcohol use disorders. Addiction 2006;101(2):212–22.

76. Campbell EJ, Lawrence AJ, Perry CJ, et al. New steps for treating alcohol use disorder. Psychopharmacology 2019;235:1759–73.

77. Martin G, Rehm J. The effectiveness of psychosocial modalities in the treatment of alcohol problems in adults: a review of the evidence. Can J Psychiatry 2012; 57(6):350–8.

78. Project MATCH Research Group. Matching alcoholism treatments to client heterogeneity: Project MATCH three-year drinking outcomes. Alcohol Clin Exp Res. 1998;22(6):1300–11.

79. Anton RF, O'Malley SS, Ciraulo DA, et al, COMBINE Study Research Group. Combined pharmacotherapies and behavioral interventions for alcohol dependence: the COMBINE study: a randomized controlled trial. JAMA 2006;295(17):2003–17.

80. Rychtarik RG, Connors GJ, Whitney RB, et al. Treatment settings for persons with alcoholism: evidence for matching clients to inpatient versus outpatient care. J Consult Clin Psychol 2000;68(2):277–89.

81. The ASAM criteria: treatment criteria for addictive, substance-related, and co-occurring conditions. In: Mee-Lee D, Shulman GD, Fishman MJ, et al, editors. The change company. 3rd edition; 2013. Carson City (NV).

82. Center for Substance Abuse Treatment. Incorporating alcohol pharmacotherapies into medical practice. Rockville (MD): Substance Abuse and Mental Health Services Administration (US); 2009 (Treatment Improvement Protocol (TIP) Series, No. 49.) Chapter 3—Disulfiram.

83. Anton RF. Naltrexone for the management of alcohol dependence. N Engl J Med 2008;359(7):715–21.

84. Maisel NC, Blodgett JC, Wilbourne PL, et al. Meta-analysis of naltrexone and acamprosate for treating alcohol use disorders: when are these medications most helpful? Addiction 2013;108(2):275–93.

85. Addolorato G, Leggio L, Ferrulli A, et al. Effectiveness and safety of baclofen for maintenance of alcohol abstinence in alcohol-dependent patients with liver cirrhosis: randomised, double-blind controlled study. Lancet 2007;370:1915–22.

86. Mason BJ, Quello S, Goodell V, et al. Gabapentin treatment for alcohol dependence: a randomized clinical trial. JAMA Intern Med 2014;174(1):70–7.

Diagnosis and Management of Opioid Use Disorder in Hospitalized Patients

Michael Herscher, MD, MA[a],*, Matthew Fine[b],
Reema Navalurkar[b], Leeza Hirt[b], Linda Wang, MD[c]

KEYWORDS

- Opioid use disorder • Hospital medicine • Inpatient management
- Substance use disorder • Heroin • Addiction • Buprenorphine • Methadone

KEY POINTS

- Despite the high rates of opioid use disorder among hospitalized patients and the availability of effective treatments, the diagnosis is often overlooked or inadequately managed during the inpatient admission.
- Opioid detoxification, a common inpatient strategy, is not effective in the treatment of opioid use disorder and is associated with increased mortality, presumably caused by loss of tolerance.
- Hospitalists should use an opioid agonist such as methadone or buprenorphine to treat acute opioid withdrawal and should offer patients continued maintenance treatment on discharge.
- Buprenorphine can be continued perioperatively and during periods of acute pain in patients already receiving it for opioid use disorder treatment.
- Hospitalists can and should play an important role in engaging patients with opioid use disorder in treatment.

BACKGROUND

Between 1999 and 2017, there were more than 702,000 deaths from drug overdose in the United States, of which 57% involved opioids.[1] This opioid overdose epidemic has taken a staggering human and economic toll, affecting men and women, most age groups, and all income levels.[1] Medications for opioid use disorder (MOUD), such as with an opioid agonist such as methadone or buprenorphine, is safe, effective, and lifesaving, but severely underused, leading to a large treatment gap.[2]

[a] Division of Hospital Medicine, Department of Medicine, Icahn School of Medicine at Mount Sinai, 1 Gustave Levy Place, New York, NY 10029, USA; [b] Department of Medical Education, Icahn School of Medicine at Mount Sinai, 1 Gustave Levy Place, New York, NY 10029, USA; [c] Division of General Internal Medicine, Department of Medicine, Icahn School of Medicine at Mount Sinai, 1 Gustave Levy Place, New York, NY 10029, USA
* Corresponding author.
E-mail address: michael.herscher@mountsinai.org

Med Clin N Am 104 (2020) 695–708
https://doi.org/10.1016/j.mcna.2020.03.003
0025-7125/20/© 2020 Elsevier Inc. All rights reserved.

medical.theclinics.com

In the context of this public health crisis, there has been an increase in hospitalizations because of the sequelae of illicit opioid use and their comorbid conditions, including endocarditis, cellulitis, osteomyelitis, and acute illness related to mental health disorders.[3,4] Opioid-related hospital admissions increased by 64% between 2005 and 2014 and an estimated 4% to 11% of hospitalized patients have opioid use disorder (OUD).[5–7] Most patients with OUD are not initiated on MOUD during hospitalization and many are not connected with outpatient treatment.[8,9] Moreover, the common strategy of opioid detoxification alone leaves patients with decreased physiologic tolerance and an increased risk for overdose on discharge.[10] Given the prevalence of OUD among hospitalized patients and opioid-related morbidity and mortality, it is incumbent on hospitalists to be familiar with the appropriate care of persons with OUD in the hospital setting.

IDENTIFYING AND DIAGNOSING OPIOID USE DISORDER IN HOSPITALIZED PATIENTS

Identifying and diagnosing OUD in hospitalized patients is the first step to providing effective intervention and evidence-based MOUD. Hospitalists should screen for illicit drug use and, if positive, conduct a nonjudgmental clinical evaluation with an in-depth history of the patient's drug use, including frequency, amount, and route of opioid administration. A formal diagnosis of OUD can be established using Diagnostic and Statistical Manual of Mental Disorders, Fifth Revision (DSM-5) criteria (**Box 1**).[11]

Despite the frequency with which patients with OUD are hospitalized for acute medical illness, physicians often fail to correctly identify and assess patients with OUD.[12] The reasons are varied, including lack of knowledge about addiction and its treatment, pessimism about its prognosis, and inaccurate beliefs regarding the legality of administering MOUD.[13] Furthermore, patients may withhold information regarding their opioid use because of fear of being judged or penalized, a consequence of deeply ingrained stigma against drug users.[14] In addition, symptoms of comorbid conditions may overlap with those indicating addiction (eg, tachycardia), or a patient's more acute medical problems may be prioritized over addressing drug use.

IDENTIFYING AND MANAGING ACUTE OPIOID WITHDRAWAL

Hospitalists should be aware of the typical presentation and time course of acute opioid withdrawal (**Table 1**).[9] Clinicians can use a validated instrument such as the Clinical Opioid Withdrawal Scale (COWS) to grade the severity of opioid withdrawal and guide therapy to reduce symptoms.[15]

The time course of opioid withdrawal depends on the opioid's half-life. For patients using short-acting opioids such as oxycodone or heroin, withdrawal symptoms typically start 8 to 12 hours after last use and peak at 36 to 72 hours. For longer-acting opioids, such as methadone, withdrawal symptoms may begin in 24 to 72 hours and peak around 4 to 6 days.[16] Unlike alcohol or benzodiazepine withdrawal, opioid withdrawal is generally not life threatening, although severe complications can occur in medically ill patients.[17]

There are several benefits to recognizing and treating opioid withdrawal in hospitalized patients. Aside from alleviating discomfort, treating withdrawal can establish trust in the clinician, providing an opportunity to treat the acute medical condition for which the patient has been hospitalized and prevent the patient from leaving against medical advice.[12] It is also a critical moment to engage the patient in maintenance OUD treatment.

In general, treatment of opioid withdrawal should include the use of opioid agonist therapy (OAT) with either methadone or buprenorphine. Studies suggest that OAT is

Box 1
Diagnostic and Statistical Manual of Mental Disorders, Fifth Revision, diagnostic criteria for opioid use disorder

A problematic pattern of opioid use leading to clinically significant impairment or distress, as manifested by at least 2 of the following, occurring within a 12-month period:
- Opioids are often taken in larger amounts or over a longer period of time than intended
- There is a persistent desire or unsuccessful efforts to cut down or control opioid use
- A great deal of time is spent in activities necessary to obtain the opioid, use the opioid, or recover from its effects
- Craving, or a strong desire to use opioids
- Recurrent opioid use resulting in failure to fulfill major role obligations at work, school, or home
- Continued opioid use despite having persistent or recurrent social or interpersonal problems caused or exacerbated by the effects of opioids
- Important social, occupational, or recreational activities are given up or reduced because of opioid use
- Recurrent opioid use in situations in which it is physically hazardous
- Continued use despite knowledge of having a persistent or recurrent physical or psychological problem that is likely to have been caused or exacerbated by opioids
- Tolerance,[a] as defined by either of the following: (1) a need for markedly increased amounts of opioids to achieve intoxication or desired effect; (2) markedly diminished effect with continued use of the same amount of an opioid
- Withdrawal,[a] as manifested by either of the following: (1) the characteristic opioid withdrawal syndrome; (2) the same (or a closely related) substance is taken to relieve or avoid withdrawal symptoms

Severity is subdivided into mild, moderate, or severe OUD:
Mild, 2 to 3 symptoms; moderate, 4 to 5 symptoms; severe, 6 or more symptoms

[a]If the opioid is being used as prescribed, this criterion is not counted toward a diagnosis of OUD.

Reprinted with permission from the Diagnostic and Statistical Manual of Mental Disorders, Fifth Edition, (Copyright ©2013). American Psychiatric Association. All Rights Reserved.

more efficacious than alpha2-adrenergic agonists such as clonidine in alleviating withdrawal symptoms and retaining patients in treatment.[18] Although clonidine is better than placebo at preventing withdrawal, it does not alleviate cravings and is generally best used in combination with OAT. Other adjunctive medications may also be helpful, including analgesics, antiemetics, antidiarrheals, and antihistamines for associated anxiety (see **Table 1**).[12]

Table 1
Common signs/symptoms and treatment of opioid withdrawal

Signs/symptoms	Treatment
Anxiety	Clonidine, diphenhydramine, hydroxyzine
Insomnia	Trazodone, diphenhydramine, hydroxyzine, melatonin
Myalgias/arthralgias/abdominal pain	Acetaminophen, ibuprofen
Diarrhea	Loperamide
Nausea/vomiting	Ondansetron

Data from TIP 63: Medications for Opioid Use Disorder – Full Document. Available at: https://medicine.yale.edu/edbup/resources/TIP_63_338482_284_42920_v1.pdf. Accessed Feb 22 2020; and Donroe JH, Holt SR, Tetrault JM. Caring for patients with opioid use disorder in the hospital. CMAJ 2016;188(17-18):1232-1239.

Both buprenorphine and methadone are similarly effective in treating opioid withdrawal.[18] In selecting between the two, providers should take into account patient needs and preferences, with a goal of discussing transition to maintenance OAT. If OAT will not be continued on discharge, methadone or buprenorphine should be tapered off over 3 to 5 days.[19]

Detoxification alone is not recommended in the treatment of OUD. Studies of patients who have undergone detoxification without continuing MOUD show an alarming relapse rate of up to 90%.[20] Treating with abstinence has also been associated with patients leaving hospitals against medical advice, as well as increased overdose risk on discharge caused by a decrease in tolerance.[21] Medically complicated and physically or emotionally distressed patients tend to respond even worse to detoxification.[14] Compared with detoxification and abstinence, MOUD is associated with reduced all-cause mortality and overdose risk and is thus the standard of care for OUD treatment.[22] Furthermore, MOUD has been shown to reduce transmission of infectious diseases such as human immunodeficiency virus (HIV) and hepatitis C, and to increase treatment retention and social functioning.[23]

INITIATING MEDICATION FOR OPIOID USE DISORDER IN THE HOSPITAL SETTING

Given the proven efficacy of MOUD, after managing acute withdrawal, clinicians should discuss maintenance treatment with the patient. Qualitative studies of hospitalized patients with substance use disorder have shown that, for many patients, hospitalization provides both a disruption in their drug use as well as a "wake-up call" about their state of health.[24] The benefits of initiating OAT before discharge have been established by several studies. In 1 randomized trial, patients with OUD who underwent inpatient buprenorphine initiation and linkage to outpatient care had decreased illicit opioid use and increased treatment retention over 6 months compared with in-hospital detoxification alone.[25] In another, hospitalized patients with OUD initiated on methadone maintenance therapy had an 82% follow-up rate at an outpatient methadone program.[26] The inpatient encounter therefore represents a so-called reachable moment in the care of patients with OUD. Hospitalists can play an important role in closing the treatment gap by approaching patients about initiating OAT with linkage to continued maintenance treatment.

MEDICATION FOR OPIOID USE DISORDER

Hospitalists should be familiar with the different options for MOUD, which include opioid agonists (methadone, buprenorphine) and an opioid antagonist (naltrexone). Although not typically an inpatient consideration, psychosocial treatment can be combined with MOUD for OUD. However, psychosocial treatment without medications may not be as effective and generally should not be offered as stand-alone therapy.[27]

Selecting the proper medication for a patient should take into account comorbid illness, risk from concurrent medications, and patient preference. A common concern related to using OAT is respiratory depression in the setting of concurrent significant alcohol or other sedating drug use. However, in 2017, the US Food and Drug Administration (FDA) recommended not withholding MOUD for patients using prescribed or illicit benzodiazepines, alcohol, or other central nervous system (CNS) depressants. Providers should instead work with patients when starting MOUD to develop strategies for safe use of prescribed or illicit benzodiazepine and CNS depressants, and tapering if appropriate.[28,29] Providers must also ensure the selected treatment is one the patient can access after discharge, and that there are available providers in the community to continue treatment. This article highlights the literature comparing the basic pharmacology, effectiveness, and clinical and legal considerations for each of these therapies.

Methadone

Pharmacology and administration

Methadone is a synthetic full opioid agonist with a variable half-life, averaging between 24 and 36 hours. It is available in liquid or tablet form and can be administered orally or by intravenous injection. Its long half-life can lead to increased risk of overdose during initial dosing and dose escalation,[12] especially when combined with other sedating agents. Adverse effects of methadone include QT interval prolongation, constipation, and respiratory depression.[30] Because it is metabolized by the liver, administration of methadone to patients with severe liver impairment should be monitored closely.[31]

Determining the proper starting dose for inpatients depends on whether the patient is already enrolled in methadone maintenance therapy (MMT). For those that are, dosing should be confirmed with the patient's methadone provider, and patients should be given their usual dose throughout the hospitalization unless there is a contraindication. For patients not enrolled in MMT, an initial dose of 10 to 30 mg should be given.[12,32] Frequent monitoring using the COWS assessment can guide subsequent dosing.[15] For patients still experiencing withdrawal, dose increases of 5 to 10 mg can be ordered as needed along with adjuvant medication for additional relief (see **Box 1**). Lower doses and slower dose titration should be used for patients at increased risk for oversedation.[9]

Clinical considerations

In the United States, outpatient MMT for OUD is highly regulated and can only be administered at an opioid treatment program (OTP), where patients must often present daily to receive their doses. Although some patients benefit from the structure of an OTP, those with variable work or family responsibilities may find accessing methadone maintenance challenging. In addition, hospitalists should be aware of the availability of treatment options in the appropriate geographic area, because there may be a paucity of OTPs in rural locations, which can be a barrier to treament.[33] Hospitalists should not initiate methadone for OUD treatment if they cannot easily follow up at an OTP, generally within 24 hours of discharge.

Although methadone is an effective choice to treat hospitalized patients' opioid addiction, administering it in the hospital setting may be underused.[34] Missed opportunities for such use may arise from physician unfamiliarity with the legality of methadone prescribing in the hospital. It is legal for hospitalists to provide methadone in the inpatient setting to patients who were admitted for reasons other than opioid detoxification or rehabilitation. Title 21 of the Code of Federal Regulations section 1306.07C does not place restrictions on using methadone to relieve acute opioid withdrawal in the hospital or initiating MOUD with the goal of continued treatment in the community after discharge.[34,35]

Buprenorphine

Pharmacology and administration

Buprenorphine is a semisynthetic opioid that is a partial agonist at the mu opioid receptor with a variable half-life of 24 to 42 hours, allowing it to be dosed daily for OUD treatment.[36] It is most commonly coformulated with naloxone in a 4:1 ratio in sublingual tablets or films. The naloxone component, added as a deterrent against intravenous administration of the drug, is inactive when buprenorphine is taken sublingually. However, if crushed or injected to be used intranasally or intravenously, naloxone exerts opioid antagonistic effects, potentially precipitating withdrawal.[37]

Because of its partial agonism, buprenorphine has a ceiling effect on respiratory depression, euphoria, and analgesia, and is normally not given at doses exceeding 24 mg/d.[9] In addition, because of its high affinity for the mu receptor, when administered in the presence of other opioids, buprenorphine displaces the other opioid from the receptor, causing a sudden decrease in receptor activation leading to abrupt withdrawal. It is therefore important that patients are in at least mild to moderate withdrawal before initiating buprenorphine, which can be determined in the hospital by waiting until the patient has a COWS score of 8 or higher. For this to occur, the authors typically wait 8 to 12 hours after last heroin or short-acting opioid use, 24 hours after a long-acting opioid (such as morphine extended release), and up to 72 hours after the last methadone use. Once the patient is in withdrawal, dosing on the first day is given in as-needed doses of 2 to 4 mg at intervals of 1 to 2 hours (**Fig. 1**) until the patient feels symptomatically improved or the COWS score is less than 8. At this point, the total dose from day 1 may be given as a daily dose beginning on day 2.[9,38]

Although adverse side effects are similar to those of other opioids, buprenorphine has a better safety profile with respect to respiratory depression, which is unlikely to occur unless combined with other sedating drugs such as benzodiazepines or alcohol. Compared with methadone, buprenorphine has not been shown to cause clinically significant QT interval prolongation.[39,40]

Clinical considerations

Unlike methadone, buprenorphine can be prescribed in an outpatient setting. Patients are given enough medication for days to months depending on the clinical scenario. Compared with no medication, office-based buprenorphine improves engagement in treatment and decreases illicit opioid use and mortality, and is cost-effective.[41,42]

Despite evidence of buprenorphine's efficacy, there exist barriers to prescribing it. Physicians, nurse practitioners, and physician's assistants must complete a training course to be granted a waiver from the FDA to prescribe buprenorphine. As of 2019, only approximately 4% of eligible physicians have obtained waivers.[43] Although policy changes have been recommended to increase access to buprenorphine, the authors believe hospitalists have an important role in expanding access to this effective treatment by initiating buprenorphine in hospitalized patients. Although a waiver is not required for clinicians to administer buprenorphine for inpatients with withdrawal,[35] we encourage hospitalists to obtain a waiver to be able to prescribe buprenorphine at discharge in order to facilitate linkage to outpatient treatment. Free waiver training can be accessed at the Providers Clinical Support System Web site: https://pcssnow.org/medication-assisted-treatment/.

Similar to methadone, hospitalists should ensure patients can follow up with a buprenorphine prescriber following discharge before initiating it in the hospital. However, because buprenorphine prescribing is less regulated than methadone, patients can follow up within 1 to 2 weeks as long as they are prescribed sufficient medication to take at home until the first outpatient visit.[9]

Naltrexone

Pharmacology and administration

Naltrexone is a competitive opioid antagonist at the mu opioid receptor, blocking the effects of opioids and thereby promoting abstinence. Naltrexone can be administered orally in daily doses or in a long-acting injectable extended-release formulation (XR-naltrexone) given once a month.[9] Although OAT with buprenorphine

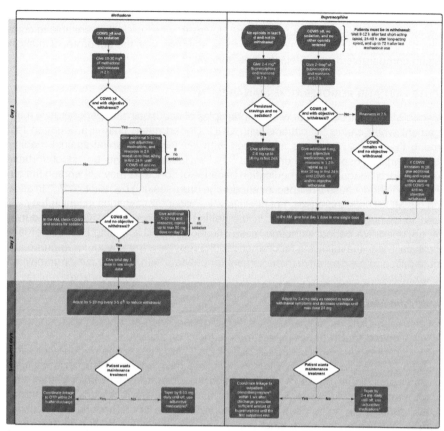

Fig. 1. Inpatient initiation of methadone and buprenorphine. [a]Give lower dose for patients at risk for oversedation (ie, older, those with respiratory disease, concurrent use of sedating medications), with no or low opioid tolerance, or who have lower daily opioid use (ie, 1–2 bags heroin per day, oxycodone 5–10 mg/d); give higher dose for patients who have higher daily opioid use/higher tolerance. Use lower dose or increase more slowly in patients who do not use opioids daily, use weaker opioids (ie, codeine), or who have not used opioids in more than 5 days. [c]Tapering off completely is associated with increased posthospital relapse and overdose; maintenance treatment is standard of care for OUD and highly encouraged. [d]This may be either a prescriber at an office-based OTP. (*Data from* Refs.[9,12,38])

or methadone is recommended as first-line treatment of moderate to severe OUD, naltrexone may be an appropriate treatment of patients with mild OUD or those who are motivated and unable to access, or unwilling to use, OAT.

When administered to individuals with recent opioid use, naltrexone can precipitate withdrawal. Therefore, patients must be opioid free for a minimum of 7 to 10 days before administering naltrexone.

Clinical considerations

The major hindrance to long-term effectiveness of oral naltrexone is adherence to daily dosing, so XR-naltrexone is preferred.[44] Another hurdle is the need to be completely abstinent before initiating naltrexone, which can be difficult for patients to tolerate. In a trial comparing XR-naltrexone with buprenorphine, 28% of patients in the naltrexone arm were unable to undergo induction and the intention-to-treat analysis found naltrexone to be inferior to buprenorphine. However, when patients were able to complete the induction, naltrexone did seem to be effective, with the per protocol analysis finding comparable rates of relapse-free survival.[45]

ACUTE PAIN AND PERIOPERATIVE MANAGEMENT

Hospitalists should be familiar with the principles of acute pain and perioperative management when caring for patients with OUD. Undertreated pain is a common fear among these patients and is associated with leaving the hospital against medical advice and in-hospital illicit drug use.[46,47] Providers may also be uncomfortable administering adequate pain medication because of concerns they will worsen the patient's addiction, cause a relapse, or encourage drug-seeking behavior.[14,48,49] In addition, as MOUD use increases, hospitalists will encounter scenarios in which they will need to manage pain medication in the setting of concomitant MOUD use during the perioperative period. Although these situations are challenging because of lack of clinical trials, the following recommendations provide a framework for approaching acute pain and perioperative management for patients with OUD who may or may not be on MOUD.

Acute Pain Management

Patients with OUD often have a physiologic dependence on opioids that requires a baseline opioid "debt" to be "repaid" before they can achieve analgesic relief. Opioid tolerance, whether from illicit opioid use or OAT with methadone or buprenorphine, must be considered before devising an adequate pain regimen. Clinicians may need to administer higher doses of opioid analgesics or more potent opioids than they would normally provide to opioid-naive patients. For patients receiving OAT, clinicians should confirm the home dose of either buprenorphine or methadone and continue this regimen. They can then either use opioid analgesics in addition to their usual buprenorphine or methadone doses, or take advantage of their intrinsic analgesic properties by increasing the dose and/or changing the frequency of administration to every 6 to 8 hours.[50]

Whenever feasible, a multimodal strategy including nonopioid analgesics and interventional pain management is recommended.[51] However, opioids are often the best analgesic option for these patients, especially in a setting of extreme pain.

Perioperative Management of Patients on Medication for Opioid Use Disorder

Patients in methadone maintenance treatment should continue taking their oral methadone on the morning of surgery and throughout the perioperative period. If they are unable to take oral medications, methadone can be given intravenously at half the usual dose. The patient's outpatient regimen is not likely to provide sufficient analgesia, therefore short-acting opioids as well as nonopioid pain medications can be given in addition to methadone to achieve adequate pain control.[52]

There is some uncertainty regarding the optimal perioperative management of patients taking buprenorphine. Given its unique pharmacologic properties, buprenorphine's high affinity for the mu opioid receptor can prevent other full opioid agonists from activating the receptor to allow additional analgesia. As a result, there is concern regarding the need to discontinue buprenorphine in order to achieve adequate postsurgical analgesia. However, this can lead to opioid withdrawal and increased risk of relapse, and existing evidence does support that maintaining buprenorphine can increase pain control while at the same time avoiding disruption of MOUD.[53–55] Thus, the emerging consensus is that, for most procedures, buprenorphine should be continued throughout the perioperative period or while the patient is having acute pain.[50,56] A dosing strategy that considers anticipated severity of postoperative pain and home buprenorphine dose can reduce the risk of withdrawal and relapse while maximizing postoperative pain management. For example, for a patient on 24mg of buprenorphine at home who is being evaluated for thoracic surgery, the provider can titrate down buprenorphine to 16mg daily on day before surgery, give 8mg on day of surgery, then 8mg daily with additional full opioid agonists as needed. [57] Similar to methadone, it can be helpful to administer buprenorphine in divided doses, 3 to 4 times per day, to take advantage of its analgesic properties.[50] Nonopioid modalities should be used when appropriate. If needed, short-acting opioids can be given, although higher doses may be required in the presence of buprenorphine. If it is determined that buprenorphine is to be stopped preoperatively, it should be slowly titrated off and held for the minimum amount of time possible (eg, 24–48 hours) to decrease the risk of relapse.[19] It should then be restarted when the patient no longer requires full opioid agonists for analgesia.

Oral naltrexone should be held for 72 hours before the procedure and XR-naltrexone should be held for at least 30 days if it is anticipated that opioids will be needed for pain control.[52]

HARM REDUCTION EDUCATION AND TECHNIQUES

It is important to approach caring for patients with OUD with harm reduction strategies in mind. All patients should be screened for HIV; latent tuberculosis; hepatitis A, B and C; and sexually transmitted infections. They should also be encouraged to receive vaccinations for hepatitis A and B if nonimmune, tetanus, and pneumonia.[58] HIV pre-exposure prophylaxis is indicated if patients have shared any injection or drug preparation equipment in the past 6 months.[59]

All patients with OUD should be given take-home naloxone, an opioid antagonist that reverses respiratory depression, before discharge.[60] Naloxone distribution has been associated with decreased overdose mortality in the community.[61]

Hospitalists should also be aware of local syringe access programs, or harm reduction organizations, and encourage patients to use their services. Providing clean needles and other drug use equipment has been shown to reduce the rates of HIV and at-risk injection practices without increasing the prevalence of drug use.[62]

DISCHARGE PLANNING

Planning for discharge and facilitating long-term follow-up care are critical when treating patients with OUD, who are at an increased risk for negative health events following discharge. One major concern is the increase in mortality after nonfatal overdose or cessation of opioids, presumably caused by loss of tolerance.[21,63] Furthermore, patients with OUD have increased rates of readmission regardless of the reason for their original hospital admission.[64] Discharge recommendations can be considered to prevent opioid overdose, prevent infection, and to link patients to ongoing care (**Table 2**).[65,66] Patients not started on MOUD can be referred to primary care as well as syringe access programs. For those started on MOUD, hospitalists should directly refer the patients to known MOUD providers in the community. Although hospital providers may not be aware of local buprenorphine-waivered physicians or OTPs, this information is readily available online, with resources such as the Substance Abuse and Mental Health Services Association's Buprenorphine

Table 2
Discharge recommendations for patients with opioid use disorder

Overdose Prevention	Infection Prevention	Linkage to Care
Provide overdose prevention education with a take-home naloxone kit to patient, family, and friends Counsel on risk reduction techniques: • Not using alone • Using rapid fentanyl test strips to detect fentanyl in drug sample • Doing a test shot to check drug potency • Have naloxone kit ready for use • Avoid using after detox or spending time in rehabilitation Avoid mixing drugs and alcohol Linkage to MOUD (buprenorphine, methadone)	Teach safe injection techniques and basic wound care Screen for HIV; hepatitis A, B, C; tuberculosis; and sexually transmitted infections Treat chronic hepatitis C infection Offer HIV preexposure prophylaxis for at-risk patients Provide vaccines for hepatitis A and hepatitis B (if nonimmune), tetanus, pneumococcus	Connect patients started on MOUD to outpatient provider/program (ie, office-based opioid treatment or opioid treatment program) Connect all patients to a primary care provider Refer to behavioral health provider for patients with co-occurring mental health disorders Refer to local syringe access programs for access to clean needles, naloxone kits, and other harm reduction resources

Data from Thakarar K, Weinstein ZM, Walley AY. Optimising health and safety of people who inject drugs during transition from acute to outpatient care: narrative review with clinical checklist. Postgrad Med J 2016;92(1088):356-363; and Harm Reduction Coalition. A Safety Manual for Injection Drug Users. Available at: https://harmreduction.org/wp-content/uploads/2011/12/getting-off-right.pdf. Accessed Feb 25 2020.

Practitioner Locator, which can be found at: https://www.samhsa.gov/medication-assisted-treatment/practitioner-program-data/treatment-practitioner-locator.

DISCLOSURE

The authors have nothing to disclose.

REFERENCES

1. Scholl L. Drug and opioid-involved overdose deaths — United States, 2013–2017. MMWR Morb Mortal Wkly Rep 2019;67. https://doi.org/10.15585/mmwr.mm6751521e1.

2. Volkow ND. Medications for opioid use disorder: bridging the gap in care. Lancet 2018;391(10118):285–7.

3. Ronan MV, Herzig SJ. Hospitalizations related to opioid abuse/dependence and associated serious infections increased sharply, 2002-12. Health Aff 2016;35(5):832–7.

4. Peterson C, Xu L, Mikosz CA, et al. US hospital discharges documenting patient opioid use disorder without opioid overdose or treatment services, 2011-2015. J Subst Abuse Treat 2018;92:35–9.

5. Weiss AJ, Elixhauser A, Barrett ML, et al. Opioid-related inpatient stays and emergency department visits by state, 2009–2014: statistical brief #219. In: Healthcare

cost and utilization project (HCUP) statistical briefs. Rockville (MD): Agency for Healthcare Research and Quality (US); 2016.

6. Holt SR, Ramos J, Harma MA, et al. Prevalence of unhealthy substance use on teaching and hospitalist medical services: implications for education. Am J Addict 2012;21(2):111–9.

7. McNeely J, Gourevitch MN, Paone D, et al. Estimating the prevalence of illicit opioid use in New York City using multiple data sources. BMC Public Health 2012;12:443.

8. Naeger S, Mutter R, Ali MM, et al. Post-discharge treatment engagement among patients with an opioid-use disorder. J Subst Abuse Treat 2016;69:64–71.

9. TIP 63: medications for opioid use disorder – full document. Available at: https://medicine.yale.edu/edbup/resources/TIP_63_338482_284_42920_v1.pdf. Accessed February 22, 2020.

10. Wines JD Jr, Saitz R, Horton NJ, et al. Overdose after detoxification: a prospective study. Drug Alcohol Depend 2007;89(2–3):161–9.

11. American Psychiatric Association. Diagnostic and statistical manual of mental disorders, fifth edition (DSM-5). Arlington (VA): American Psychiatric Association; 2013.

12. Donroe JH, Holt SR, Tetrault JM. Caring for patients with opioid use disorder in the hospital. CMAJ 2016;188(17–18):1232–9.

13. Miller NS, Sheppard LM, Colenda CC, et al. Why physicians are unprepared to treat patients who have alcohol- and drug-related disorders. Acad Med 2001;76(5):410–8.

14. Haber PS. Management of injecting drug users admitted to hospital. Lancet 2009;374(9697):1284–93.

15. Wesson DR, Ling W. The clinical opiate withdrawal scale (COWS). J Psychoactive Drugs 2003;35(2):253–9.

16. Sevarino KA. Opioid withdrawal in adults: Clinical manifestations, course, assessment, and diagnosis. In: Saxon AJ, Hermann R, editors. UpToDate. Waltham (MA): UpToDate; 2019.

17. Kosten TR, O'Connor PG. Management of drug and alcohol withdrawal. N Engl J Med 2003;348(18):1786–95.

18. Gowing L, Ali R, White JM, et al. Buprenorphine for managing opioid withdrawal. Cochrane Database Syst Rev 2017;(2):CD002025.

19. Center for Substance Abuse Treatment. Clinical guidelines for the use of buprenorphine in the treatment of opioid addiction. Rockville (MD): Substance Abuse and Mental Health Services Administration (US); 2012.

20. Smyth BP, Barry J, Keenan E, et al. Lapse and relapse following inpatient treatment of opiate dependence. Ir Med J 2010;103(6):176–9.

21. Strang J, McCambridge J, Best D, et al. Loss of tolerance and overdose mortality after inpatient opiate detoxification: follow up study. BMJ 2003;326(7396):959–60.

22. Sordo L. Mortality risk during and after opioid substitution treatment: systematic review and meta-analysis of cohort studies. BMJ 2017;357.

23. Volkow ND, Frieden TR, Hyde PS, et al. Medication-assisted therapies–tackling the opioid-overdose epidemic. N Engl J Med 2014;370(22):2063–6.

24. Velez CM, Nicolaidis C, Korthuis PT, et al. "It's been an experience, a life learning experience": a qualitative study of hospitalized patients with substance use disorders. J Gen Intern Med 2017;32(3):296–303.

25. Liebschutz JM. Buprenorphine treatment for hospitalized, opioid-dependent patients: a randomized clinical trial. JAMA Intern Med 2014;174(8):1369–76.

26. Shanahan CW, Beers D, Alford DP, et al. A transitional opioid program to engage hospitalized drug users. J Gen Intern Med 2010;25(8):803–8.

27. Blanco C, Volkow ND. Management of opioid use disorder in the USA: present status and future directions. Lancet 2019;393(10182):1760–72.

28. Center for Drug Evaluation, Research. FDA Drug Safety Communication: FDA urges caution about withholding opioid addiction medications from patients taking benzo-diazepines or CNS depressants: careful medication management can reduce risks | FDA. U.S. Food and Drug Administration. 2019. Available at: http://www.fda.gov/drugs/drug-safety-and-availability/fda-drug-safety-communication-fda-urges-caution-about-withholding-opioid-addiction-medications. Accessed November 26, 2019.

29. Martin SA, Chiodo LM, Bosse JD, et al. The next stage of buprenorphine care for opioid use disorder. Ann Intern Med 2018;169(9):628–35.

30. Chou R, Cruciani RA, Fiellin DA, et al. Methadone safety: a clinical practice guideline from the American Pain Society and College on Problems of Drug Dependence, in collaboration with the Heart Rhythm Society. J Pain 2014; 15(4):321–37.

31. UpToDate. Available at: https://www-uptodate-com.eresources.mssm.edu/contents/methadone-drug-information?search=methadone&topicRef=87238&source=see_link. Accessed December 1, 2019.

32. Kampman K, Jarvis M. American Society of Addiction Medicine (ASAM) National practice guideline for the use of medications in the treatment of addiction involving opioid use. J Addict Med 2015;9(5):358–67.

33. Johnson Q, Mund B, Joudrey PJ. Improving rural access to opioid treatment pro-grams. J Law Med Ethics 2018;46(2):437–9.

34. Noska A, Mohan A, Wakeman S, et al. Managing opioid use disorder during and after acute hospitalization: a case-based review clarifying methadone regulation for acute care settings. J Addict Behav Ther Rehabil 2015;4(2). https://doi.org/10.4172/2324-9005.1000138.

35. Winetsky D. Expanding treatment opportunities for hospitalized patients with opioid use disorders. J Hosp Med 2018;13(1):62–4.

36. Coe MA, Lofwall MR, Walsh SL. Buprenorphine pharmacology review: update on transmucosal and long-acting formulations. J Addict Med 2019;13(2):93–103.

37. Urnoski E. Why is buprenorphine coformulated with naloxone? JAAPA 2017; 30(11):44–5.

38. TOOLKIT — Project SHOUT. Project SHOUT. Available at: https://sarah-windels-b4j2.squarespace.com/toolkit. Accessed February 22, 2020.

39. Poole SA, Pecoraro A, Subramaniam G, et al. Presence or absence of QTc pro-longation in buprenorphine-naloxone among youth with opioid dependence. J Addict Med 2016;10(1):26–33.

40. Wedam EF, Bigelow GE, Johnson RE, et al. QT-interval effects of methadone, lev-omethadyl, and buprenorphine in a randomized trial. Arch Intern Med 2007; 167(22):2469–75.

41. Schackman BR, Leff JA, Polsky D, et al. Cost-effectiveness of long-term outpa-tient buprenorphine-naloxone treatment for opioid dependence in primary care. J Gen Intern Med 2012;27(6):669–76.

42. Mattick RP, Breen C, Kimber J, et al. Buprenorphine maintenance versus placebo or methadone maintenance for opioid dependence. Cochrane Database Syst Rev 2014;2:CD002207.

43. Haffajee RL, Bohnert ASB, Lagisetty PA. Policy pathways to address provider workforce barriers to buprenorphine treatment. Am J Prev Med 2018;54(6 Suppl 3):S230–42.

44. Swift R, Oslin DW, Alexander M, et al. Adherence monitoring in naltrexone pharmacotherapy trials: a systematic review. J Stud Alcohol Drugs 2011;72(6):1012–8.

45. Lee JD, Nunes EV Jr, Novo P, et al. Comparative effectiveness of extended-release naltrexone versus buprenorphine-naloxone for opioid relapse prevention (X:BOT): a multicentre, open-label, randomised controlled trial. Lancet 2018;391(10118):309–18.

46. Ti L, Voon P, Dobrer S, et al. Denial of pain medication by health care providers predicts in-hospital illicit drug use among individuals who use illicit drugs. Pain Res Manag 2015;20(2):84–8.

47. Ti L, Ti L. Leaving the hospital against medical advice among people who use illicit drugs: a systematic review. Am J Public Health 2015;105(12):e53–9.

48. Berg KM, Arnsten JH, Sacajiu G, et al. Providers' experiences treating chronic pain among opioid-dependent drug users. J Gen Intern Med 2009;24(4):482–8.

49. Baldacchino A, Gilchrist G, Fleming R, et al. Guilty until proven innocent: a qualitative study of the management of chronic non-cancer pain among patients with a history of substance abuse. Addict Behav 2010;35(3):270–2.

50. Scholzen E, Zeng AM, Schroeder KM. Perioperative management and analgesia for patients taking buprenorphine and other forms of medication-assisted treatment for substance abuse disorders. Adv Anesth 2019;37:65–86.

51. Chou R, Gordon DB, de Leon-Casasola OA, et al. Management of postoperative pain: a clinical practice guideline from the American Pain Society, the American Society of Regional Anesthesia and Pain Medicine, and the American Society of Anesthesiologists' Committee on Regional Anesthesia, Executive Committee, and Administrative Council. J Pain 2016;17(2):131–57.

52. Coluzzi F, Bifulco F, Cuomo A, et al. The challenge of perioperative pain management in opioid-tolerant patients. Ther Clin Risk Manag 2017;13:1163–73.

53. Silva MJ, Rubinstein A. Continuous perioperative sublingual buprenorphine. J Pain Palliat Care Pharmacother 2016;30(4):289–93.

54. Macintyre PE, Russell RA, Usher KAN, et al. Pain relief and opioid requirements in the first 24 hours after surgery in patients taking buprenorphine and methadone opioid substitution therapy. Anaesth Intensive Care 2013;41(2):222–30.

55. Kornfeld H, Manfredi L. Effectiveness of full agonist opioids in patients stabilized on buprenorphine undergoing major surgery: a case series. Am J Ther 2010;17(5):523–8.

56. Alford DP, Compton P, Samet JH. Acute pain management for patients receiving maintenance methadone or buprenorphine therapy. Ann Intern Med 2006;144(2):127.

57. Acampora GA, Nisavic M, Zhang Y. Perioperative Buprenorphine Continuous Maintenance and Administration Simultaneous With Full Opioid Agonist. The Journal of Clinical Psychiatry 2020;81(1).

58. Visconti AJ, Sell J, Greenblatt AD. Primary Care for Persons Who Inject Drugs. Am Fam Physician 2019;99(2):109–16.

59. US Preventive Services Task Force, Owens DK, Davidson KW, et al. Preexposure prophylaxis for the prevention of HIV infection: US preventive services task force recommendation statement. JAMA 2019;321(22):2203–13.

60. Office of the Surgeon General, Assistant Secretary for Health (ASH). U.S. Surgeon General's Advisory on Naloxone and Opioid Overdose. HHS.gov. 2018. Available at: https://www.hhs.gov/surgeongeneral/priorities/opioids-and-addiction/naloxone-advisory/index.html. Accessed December 5, 2019.

61. Walley AY, Xuan Z, Hackman HH, et al. Opioid overdose rates and implementation of overdose education and nasal naloxone distribution in Massachusetts: interrupted time series analysis. BMJ 2013;346:f174.

62. Fernandes RM, Cary M, Duarte G, et al. Effectiveness of needle and syringe programmes in people who inject drugs - An overview of systematic reviews. BMC Public Health 2017;17(1):309.

63. Larochelle MR, Bernson D, Land T, et al. Medication for opioid use disorder after nonfatal opioid overdose and association with mortality. Ann Intern Med 2018; 169(3):137.

64. Peterson C, Liu Y, Xu L, et al. U.S. National 90-day readmissions after opioid overdose discharge. Am J Prev Med 2019;56(6):875–81.

65. Thakarar K, Weinstein ZM, Walley AY. Optimising health and safety of people who inject drugs during transition from acute to outpatient care: narrative review with clinical checklist. Postgrad Med J 2016;92(1088):356–63.

66. Harm reduction coalition. A safety manual for injection drug users. Available at: https://harmreduction.org/wp-content/uploads/2011/12/getting-off-right.pdf. Accessed February 25, 2020.

Periprocedural Management of Oral Anticoagulation

Joseph R. Shaw, MD[a], Eric Kaplovitch, MD[b], James Douketis, MD, FRCP(C)[c,d,*]

KEYWORDS

- Anticoagulants • Apixaban • Atrial fibrillation • Dabigatran • Perioperative period
- Postoperative complications • Rivaroxaban • Warfarin

KEY POINTS

- Warfarin is interrupted 5 days before a procedure and can be resumed on the evening of surgery in most cases.
- Direct oral anticoagulants are interrupted 1 day before low bleed risk procedures and 2 days before high bleed risk procedures. Longer interruption intervals may be needed for patients with renal dysfunction on dabigatran.
- Direct oral anticoagulants are resumed 24 hours after low bleed risk procedures and 48 to 72 hours after high bleed risk procedures.

INTRODUCTION

Oral anticoagulation therapy is widely used for stroke prevention in patients with atrial fibrillation or mechanical heart valves, as well as for the treatment and prevention of venous thromboembolism (VTE). The need for periprocedural interruption of oral anticoagulation is therefore a commonly encountered clinical scenario. Decisions surrounding anticoagulation interruption balance the risk of excessive bleeding and thromboembolic (TE) complications. Most practitioners are familiar with vitamin K antagonists (VKAs), because they have been the most prevalent anticoagulant for the past 60 years.[1] The introduction of the direct oral anticoagulants (DOACs) over the past decade has added complexity to the periprocedural management of oral

[a] Ottawa Blood Disease Center, Division of Hematology, The Ottawa Hospital, Box 206, 501 Smyth Road, Ottawa, Ontario K1H 8L6, Canada; [b] Department of Medicine, University Health Network, The University of Toronto, 585 University Avenue, Norman Urquhart Building, 7th Floor, Room 739, Toronto, Ontario M5G 2N2, Canada; [c] Department of Medicine, Division of General Internal Medicine, McMaster University, St. Joseph's Healthcare Hamilton, 50 Charlton Avenue East, Hamilton, Ontario L4N 4A6, Canada; [d] Department of Medicine, Division of Hematology and Thromboembolism, McMaster University, St. Joseph's Healthcare Hamilton, 50 Charlton Avenue East, Hamilton, Ontario L4N 4A6, Canada
* Corresponding author. 50 Charlton Avenue East, Hamilton, Ontario L4N 4A6, Canada.
E-mail address: jdouket@mcmaster.ca
Twitter: @JRand083 (J.R.S.); @kaplovitch (E.K.)

Med Clin N Am 104 (2020) 709–726
https://doi.org/10.1016/j.mcna.2020.02.005
0025-7125/20/© 2020 Elsevier Inc. All rights reserved.
medical.theclinics.com

anticoagulants. Optimal periprocedural anticoagulation management continues to evolve. Decisions surrounding anticoagulation interruption must consider patient-specific risk of TE events, procedural risk of bleeding, pharmacokinetics of the anticoagulant in question and renal function.

PHARMACOKINETICS AND PHARMACODYNAMICS OF VITAMIN K ANTAGONISTS

VKAs, such as warfarin, make up an important yet diminishing proportion of pre-scribed oral anticoagulants.[2,3] Warfarin is the most commonly prescribed VKA in North America.[4] Warfarin has a half-life of 36 to 42 hours.[5] A 5-day interruption period before invasive procedures was originally devised using knowledge of warfarin phar-macokinetics and the time required to replenish vitamin K-dependent coagulation factors.[5,6]

Warfarin interruption protocols have been evaluated in several studies. A prospec-tive multicenter single-arm cohort study evaluating a low-molecular-weight heparin (LMWH) bridging protocol interrupted warfarin therapy 5 days preoperatively and found that only 6.7% of patients had an international normalized ratio (INR) of greater than 1.5 on the day before their procedure.[7] A randomized controlled trial evaluating different warfarin interruption protocols found that the arm involving a 5-day interrup-tion period had a mean INR of 1.2 on the day before the procedure.[8]

In general, warfarin is reinitiated either on the evening of the surgery, or the morning after, so long as patients are tolerating oral intake, no further invasive procedures are imminently planned, and hemostasis is secured. Given its indirect mechanism of ac-tion, warfarin's onset of effect is delayed by 2 to 3 days.[9] There is ongoing uncertainty surrounding the best approach to warfarin resumption after invasive procedures, although it can take up to 7 to 14 days after postoperative reinitiation of warfarin at a patient's usual maintenance dosing to attain a therapeutic INR. Studies have demonstrated that a warfarin loading dose for 2 days (defined as a doubling of pa-tients' usual warfarin maintenance dose) can achieve a faster time to therapeutic INR by 1 to 2 days and does not result in an increase in either TE or major bleeding events.[7,10]

PERIPROCEDURAL BRIDGING ANTICOAGULATION THERAPY

The pharmacokinetic properties of warfarin make it cumbersome to use in the peri-operative period. Interruption of warfarin therapy often results in upwards of 1 week of subtherapeutic anticoagulation, which may place some patients at increased risk of perioperative TE events.[10] To circumvent these limitations, perioperative bridging anticoagulation therapy with LMWH is considered. A peak therapeutic effect with LMWH occurs 3 to 5 hours after administration, with half-lives of 3 to 4 hours.[11] As a result, LMWH can be used to cover the perioperative subtherapeutic gaps created by warfarin's slow onset and offset of action. However, practices surrounding bridging therapy have changed over the past several years. A meta-analysis of 34 observational studies and randomized clinical trials totaling 12,278 patients found a pooled postoperative TE event rate of 0.9% (95% confidence interval [CI], 0.0–3.4) for patients undergoing some form of bridging therapy, compared with 0.6% (95% CI, 0.0–1.2) for patients who were not bridged.[12] No difference in the risk of TE events was found among studies comparing bridged and nonbridged groups (odds ratio [OR], 0.8; 95% CI, 0.42 to 1.54), although bridging was associated with an increased risk of overall bleeding (OR, 5.40; 95% CI, 3.00–9.74) and major bleeding (OR, 3.60; 95% CI, 1.52–8.50). The caveat to the interpretation of these data are that most of the included studies were comparative cohort studies, with control groups frequently consisting of low TE risk patients.[12] Thus, the lack of difference in postoperative TE events in this study could have been due systemic bias toward an increased baseline risk of TE events in bridged patients. This meta-analysis was followed by the BRIDGE trial, a double-blind, placebo-controlled trial comparing the perioperative interruption of warfarin therapy with and without administration of LMWH bridging in patients with atrial fibrillation.[13] The BRIDGE trial found no significant difference in rates of arterial thromboembolism between bridged and non-bridged patients of 0.3% and 0.4%, respectively, whereas there was a significant increase in major bleeding complications in the bridged group (3.2% vs 1.3%; $P = .005$). The clinical usefulness of LMWH bridging among warfarin-treated patients with atrial fibrillation or a mechanical valve was evaluated in the recently published PERIOP 2 trial.[14] This study randomized patients postoperatively to receive dalteparin bridging (prophylactic dosing if at high bleed risk, therapeutic dose if low bleed risk, based on this study's bleeding risk classification) or placebo, with all patients receiving full-dose LMWH bridging preoperatively. Among the overall study population of 1167 patients, postoperative TE and major bleeding event rates were comparable between the 2 arms. The subgroup of 304 patients with mechanical heart valves (132 mitral, 172 aortic) demonstrated no significant difference in TE events (0% vs 0.7%; $P = .50$) or major bleeding (2% vs 0.7%; $P = .62$) in bridged and non-bridged groups. The study was likely underpowered to detect such differences in patients with mechanical heart valves.

PHARMACOKINETICS, PHARMACODYNAMICS, AND PERIPROCEDURAL MANAGEMENT OF DIRECT ORAL ANTICOAGULANTS

The DOACs include the direct thrombin inhibitor dabigatran, as well as the direct Xa inhibitors rivaroxaban, apixaban, and edoxaban. DOACs have a rapid onset of action, with peak action 1 to 3 hours after intake and half-lives of 10 to 14 hours (**Table 1**).[15–19] This rapid offset and onset of action obviates the need for periprocedural bridging anticoagulation. All DOACs exhibit some degree of renal drug clearance, with dabigatran demonstrating the highest dependence on renal elimination (see **Table 1**).[20] Patients on dabigatran with renal dysfunction (creatinine clearance of <50 mL/min) require longer preprocedural DOAC interruption periods, because more time is required for drug elimination (**Fig. 1**). Based on these properties, guidance statements currently recommend that DOACs be withheld for a duration equivalent to 2 to 3 half-lives (approximately 24–36 hours) for low or moderate bleed risk procedures and 4 to 5 half-lives (approximately 48–60 hours) for high bleed risk procedures.[21]

Post hoc analyses of the pivotal trials evaluating DOAC use in atrial fibrillation have assessed outcomes after procedural interruptions.[22–25] Protocols for anticoagulation interruption generally mandated that DOACs be discontinued 2 to 3 days before invasive procedures.[26–28] In the case of dabigatran, it was being discontinued 24 hours before all procedures, irrespective of bleed risk, until the perioperative interruption protocol was modified to allow longer interruption in high bleed risk procedures.[29,30] In a meta-analysis of these retrospective studies,[31] no difference was found when comparing postoperative outcomes between patients on warfarin and DOACs. The pooled 30-day postoperative major bleeding rate of patients on DOACs was 1.81% (95% CI, 0.84–3.1), which is comparable with the rates of major bleeding in studies of perioperative VKA management.[13] These retrospective perioperative analyses have several limitations that limit their clinical applicability: perioperative DOAC interruption and resumption were not standardized, procedural bleed risk stratification was not incorporated into the perioperative anticoagulation management,[26,32] there was

Table 1
DOAC pharmacokinetic/pharmacodynamic properties

| Pharmacokinetics/Pharmacodynamics | DOAC | | | |
	Dabigatran (Pradaxa)	Rivaroxaban (Xarelto)	Apixaban (Eliquis)	Edoxaban (Savaysa/Lixiana)
Time to peak concentration (C_{max}, hours)	1–2	2–4	3–4	1–2
Half-life ($t_{1/2}$, hours)	12–17	5–13	12	10–14
Renal elimination (%)	80	35	27	50
Recommended DOAC assay – most sensitive	Thrombin Time	Calibrated anti-Xa	Calibrated anti-Xa	Calibrated anti-Xa
Recommended DOAC assay - correlation with drug levels	Dilute thrombin time/aPTT[a]	Calibrated anti-Xa	Calibrated anti-Xa	Calibrated anti-Xa
Expected range of plasma levels at peak for standard dose (ng/mL)	64–443	184–343	69–321	91–321
Expected range of plasma levels at trough for standard dose (ng/mL)	31–225	12–137	34–230	31–230

[a] aPTT testing demonstrates reasonable correlation with dabigatran levels and is more widely available as compared with dilute thrombin time. aPTT assay sensitivity is reagent and assay-dependent. A normal aPTT does not rule out the presence of "on-therapy" dabigatran levels.

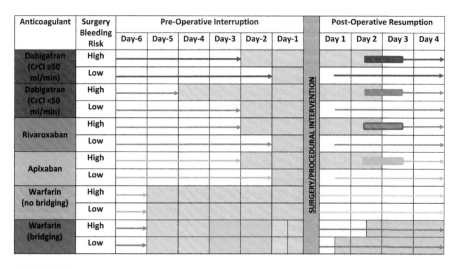

Anticoagulant	Surgery Bleeding Risk	Pre-Operative Interruption							Post-Operative Resumption			
		Day-6	Day-5	Day-4	Day-3	Day-2	Day-1		Day 1	Day 2	Day 3	Day 4
Dabigatran (CrCl ≥50 ml/min)	High											
	Low											
Dabigatran (CrCl <50 ml/min)	High											
	Low											
Rivaroxaban	High											
	Low											
Apixaban	High											
	Low											
Warfarin (no bridging)	High											
	Low											
Warfarin (bridging)	High											
	Low											

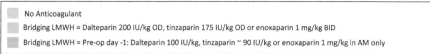

No Anticoagulant

Bridging LMWH = Dalteparin 200 IU/kg OD, tinzaparin 175 IU/kg OD or enoxaparin 1 mg/kg BID

Bridging LMWH = Pre-op day -1: Dalteparin 100 IU/kg, tinzaparin ~ 90 IU/kg or enoxaparin 1 mg/kg in AM only

Fig. 1. VKA/DOAC anticoagulation interruption.

an under-representation of patients undergoing major surgery, and perioperative bridging anticoagulation was allowed at the treating physician's discretion.[26,27] These studies therefore provide support that preoperative interruption of DOACs 2 to 4 days before surgery is associated with low postoperative event rates, although extrapolation of these results to contemporary interruption practices may be hindered owing to these limitations.

THE ROLE OF DIRECT ORAL ANTICOAGULANT LABORATORY TESTING IN THE PERIOPERATIVE SETTING

The role of laboratory testing for DOACs in clinical practice, in general, and in the perioperative setting is uncertain. DOAC testing is not widely available and the interpretation of DOAC levels is not standardized. For dabigatran, the thrombin time is highly sensitive to dabigatran levels, and a normal thrombin time is associated with no dabigatran anticoagulant effect (see **Table 1**).[33] The dilute thrombin time, expressed as nanograms per milliliter, seems to correlate well with dabigatran levels.[34] The activated partial thromboplastin time (aPTT) has some correlation with dabigatran levels, although this seems to be the case with more sensitive aPTT assays.[35] A normal aPTT may exclude above on-therapy levels of dabigatran but may not be sufficiently sensitive to exclude a clinically important anticoagulant level. For the oral Xa inhibitors, the prothrombin time and aPTT demonstrate variable and unreliable sensitivity to detect DOAC levels.[35,36] Rivaroxaban, and to a lesser extent, edoxaban, may affect the prothrombin time, but the prothrombin time is insensitive to the effects of apixaban. Generally, calibrated anti-Xa chromogenic assays using DOAC-specific calibrators are sensitive and seem to be the best method to measure oral Xa inhibitor levels. With respect to elective surgery, preprocedural coagulation testing for patients on DOAC therapy is generally not recommended. There is ongoing debate as to the role of DOAC level laboratory testing in the perioperative setting.[37,38] Current DOAC level thresholds to allow surgery are empiric, based on pharmacokinetic considerations[39] and lower limits of DOAC level detection.[40]

Prospective cohort studies have measured residual preoperative DOAC levels following standardized perioperative DOAC interruption protocols based on pharmacokinetic principles and procedural bleeding risk. CORIDA was a prospective, 422-patient, multicenter registry study where DOAC levels were measured preprocedure with the goal of identifying factors that influence residual DOAC levels.[41] The timing of DOAC interruption was at the discretion of the treating clinician, with a median duration of DOAC interruption of 66 hours (range, 1–218 hours). Preprocedural DOAC levels ranged from 30 ng/mL or less to 527 ng/mL; 77% of patients had levels of 30 ng/mL or less, and 86% had levels of 50 ng/mL or less. Among patients with an interruption interval of 25 to 48 hours, 38% had DOAC levels of 30 ng/mL or greater and approximately 20% had 50 ng/mL or greater, although most of these patients had interruptions intervals closer to 24 than 48 hours. Only 5% of patients with an interruption of 49 hours or more had DOAC levels of 30 ng/mL or greater, and none had levels of 50 ng/mL or greater.

The PAUSE trial[42] was a prospective multicenter cohort study that evaluated a standardized perioperative management strategy in DOAC-treated patients with atrial fibrillation who required an elective surgery or procedure. The perioperative DOAC interruption and resumption approach was anchored on DOAC-specific pharmacokinetic properties, procedure-associated bleeding risk, and patient renal function.[12,13] DOACs were omitted for 1 day before and 1 day after low bleed risk surgery/procedures (corresponding with a 30- to 36-hour interruption interval) and for 2 days before and 2 days after a high bleed risk surgery or procedure (corresponding with a 60- to 68-hour interruption interval). For dabigatran-treated patients with a creatinine clearance of 50 mL/min or less, an additional 1 or 2 days of interruption was added to account for dabigatran's renal dependence on clearance. DOACs were resumed approximately 24 hours after low bleed risk procedures and approximately 48 to 72 hours after high bleed risk procedures. For clarification, in the PAUSE study report, a low bleed risk surgery or procedure equates with a low or moderate bleed risk surgery or procedure as defined by the recent International Society on Thrombosis and Haemostasis (ISTH) surgery or procedure bleed risk classification. The $CHADS_2$ score was not incorporated into periprocedural decision making, given that the associated TE risk primarily influences the decision to use therapeutic bridging anticoagulation in warfarin-treated patients. Patients deemed at high risk of postoperative VTE events could receive prophylactic dose heparin if patients could not take oral medications. Overall, the 30-day postoperative rate of major bleeding rate was 1.35% (95% CI, 0%–2.00%) in the apixaban cohort, 0.90% (95% CI, 0%–1.73%) in the dabigatran cohort and 1.85% (95% CI, 0%–2.65%) in the rivaroxaban cohort. Among the 85% of patients who had DOAC levels just before the surgery or procedure, the proportions of patients with levels of 50 ng/mL or less were 90.5%, 95.1% and 96.8% in the apixaban, dabigatran, and rivaroxaban cohorts, respectively. Among patients having a high bleed risk procedure, 98.8% had DOAC levels of less than 50 ng/mL. The proportion of patients undergoing high bleed risk procedures on apixaban, dabigatran, and rivaroxaban with residual levels of 30 to 49.9 ng/mL was 4.80%, 0.55%, and 14.00%, respectively. The rates of perioperative major bleeding in PAUSE are comparable with those in a prospective cohort study of dabigatran (1.8%; 95% CI, 0.7–3.0),[43] a registry of nonstandardized perioperative DOAC management (1.2%, 95% CI, 0.6–2.1),[44] and a meta-analysis (1.81%; 95% CI, 0.84–3.1).[31]

NEURAXIAL ANESTHESIA
Vitamin K Antagonists

All procedures involving neuraxial anesthesia are managed as high bleeding risk procedures, given the serious consequences of neuraxial bleeding.[6] Preoperative management of warfarin in patients receiving neuraxial anesthesia follows the same approach as in other patients with the caveat that measurement of the INR on preoperative day 1 may be done to ensure a normalized or near-normalized INR and provides the opportunity to administer low-dose (1–2 mg) oral vitamin K in the event of an INR of 1.5 or greater.[45,46]

Postoperatively, warfarin is resumed after the epidural catheter is removed, whether patients receive neuraxial anesthesia alone or neuraxial anesthesia followed by continuous epidural analgesia. If patients are to receive LMWH bridging, this therapy should be initiated after removal of the epidural catheter. However, low-dose LMWH can be co-administered with continuous epidural analgesia.[47]

Direct Oral Anticoagulants

Data on the interruption and resumption of DOAC therapy is sparse in patients undergoing neuraxial procedures. The 2018 American Society of Regional Anesthesia guidelines recommend apixaban and rivaroxaban discontinuation at least 72 hours before a neuraxial procedure.[45] In the PAUSE study, the median interruption interval for patients having a high bleed risk surgery/procedure, which encompassed any neuraxial intervention was 63.8 hours for patients taking apixaban and 72 hours for those taking rivaroxaban.[42] The American Society of Regional Anesthesia recommends dabigatran to be discontinued 72 to 120 hours before a neuraxial procedure, depending on patient creatinine clearance. In the PAUSE study, the median interval was 63.2 hours for patients with a creatinine clearance of greater than 50 mL/min and 110.2 hours for those with a creatinine clearance of less than 50 mL/min.

Postoperatively, the American Society of Regional Anesthesia recommends resumption of DOACs 24 hours after surgery and removal of the epidural catheter or end of the neuraxial procedure. In the PAUSE study, resumption of DOACs after the removal of the epidural catheter or end of the neuraxial procedure was based on the procedure-associated bleed risk: 24 hours for low bleed risk; 48 to 72 hours for high bleed risk.

THROMBOEMBOLIC RISK STRATIFICATION

A key component of a periprocedural management plan involves stratification of a patient's TE risk and procedural bleed risk (**Table 2**). TE risk stratification schemes are rough approximations based on annual stroke rates, not based on true periprocedural stroke rates. For this reason, these stratification schemes should be used as guides only, and should not supersede clinical judgment. Stratification in the current era of perioperative anticoagulation management serves mainly to identify patients on VKA therapy at high risk of TE events who may derive benefit from therapeutic bridging anticoagulation, although there is mounting evidence that bridging anticoagulation does not reduce the risk of postoperative TE events.[13,14] Because bridging therapy is not needed in DOAC-treated patients, TE risk stratification should not influence periprocedural management of such patients.[42]

Bridging anticoagulation should be considered in selected patients, including those with mechanical mitral valves (see **Table 2**), older tilting disc valves in mitral/aortic positions, patients with atrial fibrillation with a recent (within 3 months) stroke, or patients with a $CHADS_2$ score of 5 to 6.[6] It remains unclear whether patients classified as high

Table 2
TE risk stratification

Risk Category	Mechanical Heart Valve	Atrial Fibrillation	VTE
High >10% risk of ATE per year -or- >10% risk of VTE per month	Mechanical mitral valve Caged ball/tilting disc mitral/aortic valve Stroke <3 mo	$CHADS_2$ = 5–6 CHA_2DS_2Vasc score ≥ 7 Stroke/TIA <3 mo Rheumatic valvular heart disease	VTE within <3 mo Protein C, protein S, or antithrombin deficiency Multiple thrombophilias VTE associated with IVC filter Cancer-associated VTE[a]
Moderate 4%–10% risk of ATE per year -or- 4%–10% risk of VTE per month	Bileaflet AVR with major risk factors for stroke (atrial fibrillation or any of the CHADS2 components)	CHADS2 = 3–4 CHA_2DS_2Vasc score = 5–6	VTE within 3–12 mo Recurrent VTE Heterozygous factor V Leiden, heterozygous prothrombin gene mutation Active cancer or recent history of cancer (within 5 y if history of cancer, excluding nonmelanomatous skin cancer)
Low <4% risk of ATE per year -or- <2% risk of VTE per month	Bileaflet AVR without major risk factors for stroke (no atrial fibrillation or none of the CHADS2 components)	$CHADS_2$ = 0–2 CHA_2DS_2Vasc = 1–4	VTE within >12 mo

Abbreviations: AVR, aortic valve replacement; IVC, inferior vena cava; TIA, transient ischemic attack.

[a] Pancreatic cancer, myeloproliferative neoplasm, glioblastoma multiforme, gastric cancer.

Adapted from Douketis JD, Spyropoulos AC, Spencer FA, et al. Perioperative management of antithrombotic therapy: Antithrombotic Therapy and Prevention of Thrombosis, 9th ed: American College of Chest Physicians Evidence-Based Clinical Practice Guidelines. Chest 2012;141(2 Suppl):e326S-e350S; and Spyropoulos AC, Brohi K, Caprini J, et al. Scientific and Standardization Committee Communication: Guidance document on the periprocedural management of patients on chronic oral anticoagulant therapy: Recommendations for standardized reporting of procedural/surgical bleed risk and patient-specific thromboembolic risk. J Thromb Haemost 2019;17(11):1966-1972; with permission.

risk truly derive benefit from bridging anticoagulation, although the results of the PERIOP2 trial suggest that some patients with mechanical valves undergoing periprocedural interruption without postoperative bridging may experience TE events at similar rates as non–high-risk patients. Definitive conclusions cannot be drawn from PERIOP2, because all patients received preoperative therapeutic bridging therapy and sample sizes were small.[14]

There is limited evidence surrounding periprocedural anticoagulation management in patients with VTE.[48–50] As with atrial fibrillation, TE risk stratification for VTE is derived from nonperioperative studies. Few studies have investigated therapeutic dose bridging in patients with VTE. One retrospective cohort study demonstrated that use of postoperative prophylactic dose LMWH in patients undergoing perioperative interruption of VKA therapy without recent (within 3 months) VTE was associated with a low rate of postoperative VTE (0.32%; 95% CI, 0.087–1.14).[48] Another retrospective cohort study of 1178 patients evaluated recurrent VTE and bleeding rates after warfarin interruption for invasive procedures in patients anticoagulated for VTE,[50] and analyzed results according to whether patients received bridging therapy or not. Patients were classified as low, moderate, or high risk for VTE, based on American College of Chest Physicians guidelines,[6] in 79.0%, 17.9%, and 3.1% of procedural interruptions, respectively. There was no difference in recurrent VTE rates among the bridging versus no-bridging groups, and no recurrent postoperative VTE occurred among high-risk patients. Bridging therapy was associated with a statistically significant increase in major bleeding (2.2% vs 0.2%; $P<.001$). Based on these results, it is reasonable to consider bridging in select patients considered to be at very high risk of VTE (ie, VTE within the last 3 months), more so owing to a lack of evidence of the safety of forgoing bridging, rather than evidence supporting the efficacy of this practice.

PROCEDURAL BLEEDING RISK STRATIFICATION

There is no standardized surgery- or procedure-related bleeding stratification scheme.[13,43,51] Bleeding risk can be classified using a 2-tiered (standard or high)[43] or 3-tiered (minimal, low, and high) scheme.[52] The 3-tiered bleeding risk stratification scheme proposed by the ISTH[21,52] (**Table 3**) directs management based on each risk group and is based on rates of postprocedural bleeding. Procedures classified as minimal bleeding risk are associated with a negligible (approximately 0%) rate of major bleeding postprocedurally, procedures classified as low bleeding risk have a less than 2% rate of major bleeding at 30 days postprocedurally and patients classified as high bleeding risk have major bleeding rates of greater than 2%. Overall, surgery- or procedure-related bleeding risk stratification is based on limited data, typically from case series and observational studies, and often with divergent definitions of major bleeding.[6,21,52] Additional multidisciplinary collaboration is needed to attain consensus on a bleed risk classification scheme according to the type of surgery or procedure.

Minimal Bleeding Risk Procedures

Patients undergoing minimal bleed risk procedures (see **Table 3**) can likely undergo procedural intervention without interruption of warfarin or DOAC therapy. This approach is supported by high-quality data with respect to pacemaker insertion[53,54] and catheter ablation of atrial fibrillation,[55] although trials evaluating the continuation of warfarin usually compared a continuation strategy with LMWH bridging and not with interruption without bridging. It is unclear whether excess bleeding would be seen if continued warfarin use were compared with warfarin interruption without bridging,

Table 3
Procedural bleeding risk stratification

Minimal Risk	Low Risk	High Risk
Minor dermatologic procedures (basal cell carcinoma/squamous cell carcinoma excisions, excision of actinic keratoses, excision of premalignant or cancerous nevi)	Arthroscopy	Any major surgery >45 min in duration
	Cutaneous biopsies	Any surgery involving neuraxial anesthesia
	Lymph node biopsies	Major surgery with planned extensive tissue injury
	Foot/hand surgery	Cancer surgery, especially solid tumor resection
	Coronary angiography[a]	Major orthopedic surgery, including shoulder replacement surgery
	Gastrointestinal endoscopy ± biopsy	Reconstructive plastic surgery
Cataract surgery	Colonoscopy ± biopsy	Urologic surgery (including TURP, TURBT, or tumor ablation, nephrectomy, kidney biopsy)
Minor dental procedures (dental extractions, restorations, prosthetics, endodontics), dental cleanings, fillings	Abdominal hysterectomy	
	Laparoscopic cholecystectomy	Gastrointestinal surgery, especially involving bowel anastomoses (including bowel resection)
	Abdominal hernia repair	Colonic polyp resection (if unknown at the time of periprocedural planning, colonoscopies should be considered high risk)
Pacemaker or ICD implantation	Hemorrhoidal surgery	
	Bronchoscopy ± biopsy	PEG placement, ERCP
Arthrocentesis or joint injection	Epidural injections	Surgery/biopsies involving highly vascular organs (kidneys, liver, spleen)
		Cardiac surgery
		Neurosurgery
		Spinal surgery

Abbreviations: ERCP, endoscopic retrograde cholangiopancreatography; ICD, implantable cardioverter-defibrillator; PEG, percutaneous endoscopic gastrostomy; TURBT, transurethral resection of bladder tumor; TURP, transurethral resection of prostate.

[a] Radial approach may be considered minimal bleeding risk compared with a femoral approach.

Adapted from Spyropoulos AC, Al-Badri A, Sherwood MW, et al. Periprocedural management of patients receiving a vitamin K antagonist or a direct oral anticoagulant requiring an elective procedure or surgery. J Thromb Haemost 2016;14(5):875-885; and Spyropoulos AC, Brohi K, Caprini J, et al. Scientific and Standardization Committee Communication: Guidance document on the periprocedural management of patients on chronic oral anticoagulant therapy: Recommendations for standardized reporting of procedural/surgical bleed risk and patient-specific thromboembolic risk. J Thromb Haemost 2019;17(11):1966-1972; with permission.

which would now be the standard of care for most patients.[13,56] The BRUISE CONTROL-2 trial demonstrated that continued use of DOAC therapy as compared with DOAC interruption was not associated with a difference in hematomas after pacemaker implantation.[54] Observational data support the safety of warfarin continuation in patients undergoing percutaneous coronary intervention, although most comparisons were with patients undergoing warfarin interruption with LMWH bridging.[57]

Numerous studies have evaluated various strategies surrounding the management of VKA therapy for dental procedures,[6] including partial (2–3 days) VKA interruption or continued VKA use with or without postprocedural administration of topical tranexamic acid.[58] There is limited evidence supporting either discontinuation or continuation of DOAC therapy for dental procedures.[59] Ambient practice is to continue anticoagulation for minor dental procedures, including restorations, prosthetics, dental extractions (1–2 teeth), endodontics (apicoectomy, root canal, implants, etc), soft tissue biopsies, cleanings, and fillings.[6,21] Although a small residual risk of bleeding exists, local strategies including absorbable sponges, oxidized cellulose, fibrin glue, suturing, and cautery, as well as local tranexamic acid, can minimize this risk further.[60]

Evidence surrounding continuation of anticoagulation in dermatologic procedures is derived from lower quality observational studies. Bleeding events in these studies were more common on continued VKA therapy. These bleeding events were generally minor and could be controlled with local hemostatic measures. Some of these studies did demonstrate that visible bleeding was increased during procedures when warfarin was continued.[61–63] A systematic review assessed the safety of continued warfarin therapy in patients undergoing cataract surgery.[64] Patients who continued warfarin had an increased risk for bleeding (OR, 3.26; 95% CI, 1.73–6.16), and the overall incidence of bleeding was 10%. Virtually all bleeding events were self-limited and minor in nature (ie, dot hyphemae, subconjunctival hemorrhage). In minor dermatologic procedures and cataract surgery, given the minimal residual bleeding risk, it is reasonable to continue anticoagulation without interruption.

Low or Moderate and High Bleeding Risk Procedures

Low or moderate and high bleed risk procedures, as classified by the ISTH, are outlined in **Table 3**.[52] Surgery lasting more than 45 minutes, any procedures involving neuraxial anesthesia, urologic surgery, major gastrointestinal surgery, surgery in highly vascular organs (kidneys, liver, spleen), and cardiac, neurosurgical, or spinal surgery are all considered high bleed risk procedures.

There have been numerous studies evaluating postprocedural bleeding rates in patients undergoing gastrointestinal endoscopic procedures.[65] The European Society of Gastrointestinal Endoscopy/British Society Gastroenterology issue recommendations for periendoscopic antithrombotic management and procedural-related bleed risk stratification.[65] Diagnostic procedures with or without biopsy, biliary or pancreatic stenting, and device-assisted enteroscopy (eg, balloon enteroscopy) are considered, based on their bleeding risk classification, as a low bleed risk, whereas any polypectomy, endoscopic retrograde cholangiopancreatography with sphincterotomy, ampullectomy, endoscopic dilation, or enteral stenting and endoscopic hemostasis are all considered high bleed risk procedures. However, these recommendations are based on data from patients who were not anticoagulated. A retrospective study of patients on continued warfarin therapy undergoing polypectomy found that 0.8% of patients had bleeding severe enough to require transfusion.[66] A randomized trial that evaluated hot (with cautery) versus cold (without cautery) snaring of polyps in anticoagulated patients found rates of immediate bleeding of 23% and 5.7%, respectively and delayed bleeding of 14% and 0%, respectively.[67] No studies have evaluated the safety of continued DOAC therapy in patients undergoing endoscopic therapies. The European Society of Gastrointestinal Endoscopy/British Society Gastroenterology guidelines recommend that patients undergoing low bleed risk procedures continue VKA therapy, whereas patients on DOACs should omit the dose on the morning of the procedure. This is in contrast with the ISTH guidance, which classifies all endoscopic procedures as either low to moderate or high bleed risk procedures (see **Table 3**), and thus would necessitate anticoagulation interruption for all

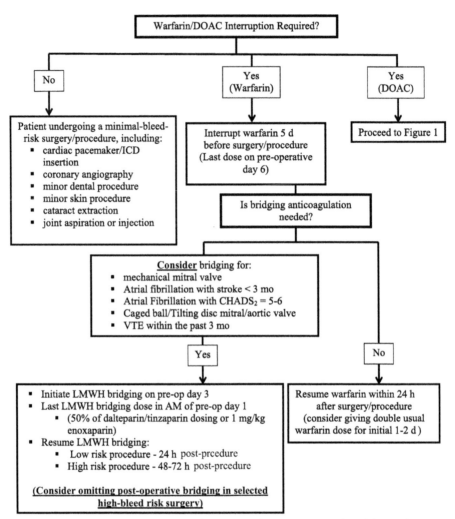

Fig. 2. Perioperative management of anticoagulants. ICD, implantable cardioverter-defibrillator.

endoscopic procedures (**Fig. 2**). The European Society of Gastrointestinal Endoscopy/British Society Gastroenterology recommendations[65] for high bleed risk procedures are consistent with those issued by ISTH.[52] There is a need for collaboration between gastroenterology- and thrombosis-based societies to develop a harmonized system of bleeding risk classification for gastrointestinal procedures and this effort is in progress.

A PRACTICAL APPROACH TO PERIPROCEDURAL ANTICOAGULATION MANAGEMENT

Perioperative VKA management incorporates patient TE and procedural bleed risk. DOAC management depends on procedural bleeding risk, pharmacokinetics, and a patient's renal function. The suggested management is consistent with ISTH guidance (see **Fig. 2**):

Box 1
St. Joseph's Healthcare contact information

905-522-1234

Dr Green/Dr Black/Dr Orange/Dr Blue– ext. 12345

Dr Red – ext. 23456 Dr Pink - ext. 34567

May or June, nurse practitioners, thrombosis - ext. 12345 or ext. 56789

Weekend thrombosis assistance: ext. 77777 ask for hematologist on call to be paged.

Emergencies report to the nearest hospital.

- Patients undergoing minimal bleed risk procedures generally do not require VKA or DOAC interruption, with the caveat that a single DOAC dose on the morning of the procedure can be omitted to avoid peak DOAC levels at the time of the procedure.
- Patients undergoing low bleed risk procedures require anticoagulant interruption. Warfarin is held for 5 days preoperatively (ie, last dose on preoperative day 6), whereas DOACs are held for 1 day preoperatively (ie, last dose on preoperative day 2). This strategy allows for 36 to 48 hours between the last dose of a DOAC and the procedure, which approximates an interval of 3 DOAC half-lives. Warfarin (and bridging therapy, if implemented) and DOACs can be resumed within 24 hours after the procedure. Warfarin is generally reinitiated the evening of the procedure and bridging therapy or DOAC therapy is reinitiated 24 hours after the procedure.
- For patients undergoing high bleed risk procedures, VKAs are held for 5 days preoperatively (ie, last dose on preoperative day 6), whereas DOACs are held for 2 days (ie, last dose on preoperative day 3). For patients taking VKAs, checking an INR on preoperative day 1 and administering 1.0 to 2.5 mg of oral vitamin K if the INR is greater than 1.5 is recommended.[46] The resumption of therapeutic anticoagulation should be delayed by 48 to 72 hours after all high-risk procedures. This means that bridging therapeutic LMWH or unfractionated heparin (in the case of VKA patients) and DOAC resumption should be delayed until postoperative days 2 to 3. Given the onset of action for DOACs is on the order of 1 to 4 hours, it is very important for clinicians to understand that full anticoagulant effect will be immediate, and thus resumption after high bleed risk procedures needs to be delayed by 48 to 72 hours. VKA therapy can often be resumed within 24 hours of high-risk procedures owing to its delayed onset of action. Careful

---

Table 4
Perioperative bridging anticoagulation program St. Joseph's Healthcare, Hamilton

Patient Name	John Doe	Today's Date	August 9, 2019
Referring MD	H. Specialist	ID:	123456
Family MD	F. Doctor	DOB:	01/01/1940
Health card #	123456789	INR Lab:	N/A
Telephone #	905-123-4567	Allergies:	NKDA
Date of surgery/procedure		August 21, 2019 – Colonoscopy	
Rivaroxaban (Xarelto):		20 mg daily @ 0830	

Abbreviations: DOB, date of birth; NKDA, no known drug allergies.

Table 5
Anticoagulation before and after the operations

Date	Days to Procedure	Action
Sunday, August 19, 2019	−2	Last dose of rivaroxaban
Monday, August 20, 2019	−1	
Tuesday, August 21, 2019	Procedure	
Wednesday, August 22, 2019	1	Restart rivaroxaban if no biopsy and no polyp removed
Thursday, August 23, 2019	2	
Friday, August 24, 2019	3	Restart rivaroxaban if biopsy taken or polyp removed

consideration should always be given to postprocedural hemostasis when resuming therapeutic anticoagulation after high bleed risk procedures. Therapeutic anticoagulation should not be resumed until adequate hemostasis has been achieved and should be delayed until neuraxial anesthesia has been discontinued.

- For patients on a VKA who are deemed to require bridging LMWH anticoagulation (see **Fig. 2**), bridging therapy is generally initiated on preoperative day 3. Therapeutic dosing (dalteparin 200 IU/kg/d, tinzaparin 175 IU/kg/d, enoxaparin 1 mg/kg twice daily) is given on preoperative days 3 and 2. A reduced dose of bridging is administered on the morning of preoperative day 1. If the patient is on twice daily dosing of enoxaparin, the same dose (1 mg/kg) can be given on the morning of preoperative day 1. If dalteparin or tinzaparin are used, 50% of the total daily dose should be given on the morning of preoperative day 1.
- A loading warfarin dose, consisting of double the patient's usual daily maintenance dose can be considered on postoperative days 1 and 2, based on evidence this achieves therapeutic INR values more rapidly without excess bleeding or thrombosis.[7,10] This may not apply to patients who are severely ill, have newly decreased oral intake (particularly after bowel surgery), or are initiated on new medications known to elevate INR (such as broad-spectrum antibiotics).

Perioperative anticoagulation management plans can be complex and difficult to understand by patients and their health care providers. As such, we recommend that a perioperative anticoagulation calendar be provided to both the patient and the consulting surgical team (**Box 1**, **Tables 4** and **5**). This increases the likelihood that patients will interrupt their anticoagulation according to the desired schedule and, in selected patients, will self-administer bridging therapy as prescribed. In addition, we encourage clear language when describing interruption intervals. It is often helpful to describe preprocedural interruptions using both the number of days off anticoagulation and the day on which the last dose of anticoagulation should be taken (eg, hold anticoagulation for 2 days preprocedurally, last dose on preoperative day 3).

DISCLOSURE

J.R. Shaw and E. Kaplovitch have no conflicts of interest to disclose. J. Douketis has received personal fees from Janssen, Pfizer, Bayer, Bristol Myers Squibb, Sanofi, Servier Canada, and Portola Pharmaceuticals.

REFERENCES

1. Witt DM, Clark NP, Kaatz S, et al. Guidance for the practical management of warfarin therapy in the treatment of venous thromboembolism. J Thromb Thrombolysis 2016;41(1):187–205.
2. Weitz JI, Semchuk W, Turpie AG, et al. Trends in prescribing oral anticoagulants in Canada, 2008-2014. Clin Ther 2015;37(11):2506–14.e4.
3. Barnes GD, Lucas E, Alexander GC, et al. National trends in ambulatory oral anticoagulant use. Am J Med 2015;128(12):1300–5.e2.
4. Pengo V, Pegoraro C, Cucchini U, et al. Worldwide management of oral anticoagulant therapy: the ISAM study. J Thromb Thrombolysis 2006;21(1):73–7.
5. Ansell J, Hirsh J, Hylek E, et al. Pharmacology and management of the vitamin K antagonists: American College of Chest Physicians Evidence-Based Clinical Practice Guidelines (8th Edition). Chest 2008;133(6 Suppl):160S–98S.
6. Douketis JD, Spyropoulos AC, Spencer FA, et al. Perioperative management of antithrombotic therapy: antithrombotic therapy and prevention of thrombosis, 9th ed: American College of Chest Physicians Evidence-Based Clinical Practice Guidelines. Chest 2012;141(2 Suppl):e326S–50S.
7. Kovacs MJ, Kearon C, Rodger M, et al. Single-arm study of bridging therapy with low-molecular-weight heparin for patients at risk of arterial embolism who require temporary interruption of warfarin. Circulation 2004;110(12):1658–63.
8. Steib A, Barre J, Mertes M, et al. Can oral vitamin K before elective surgery substitute for preoperative heparin bridging in patients on vitamin K antagonists? J Thromb Haemost 2010;8(3):499–503.
9. Palareti G, Legnani C. Warfarin withdrawal. Pharmacokinetic-pharmacodynamic considerations. Clin Pharmacokinet 1996;30(4):300–13.
10. Schulman S, Hwang HG, Eikelboom JW, et al. Loading dose vs. maintenance dose of warfarin for reinitiation after invasive procedures: a randomized trial. J Thromb Haemost 2014;12(8):1254–9.
11. Garcia DA, Baglin TP, Weitz JI, et al. Parenteral anticoagulants: antithrombotic therapy and prevention of thrombosis, 9th ed: American College of Chest Physicians Evidence-Based Clinical Practice Guidelines. Chest 2012;141(2 Suppl):e24S–43S.
12. Siegal D, Yudin J, Kaatz S, et al. Periprocedural heparin bridging in patients receiving vitamin K antagonists: systematic review and meta-analysis of bleeding and thromboembolic rates. Circulation 2012;126(13):1630–9.
13. Douketis JD, Spyropoulos AC, Kaatz S, et al. Perioperative bridging anticoagulation in patients with atrial fibrillation. N Engl J Med 2015;373(9):823–33.
14. Kovacs M, Rodger M, Wells P, et al. Double blind randomized control trial of postoperative low molecular weight heparin bridging therapy for patients who are at high risk for arterial thromboembolism (PERIOP 2). Blood 2018;132:424.
15. Xarelto (rivaroxaban). Titusville (NJ): Janssen Pharmaceuticals LLC; 2019.
16. Eliquis (apixaban). Princeton (NJ): Bristol-Myers Squibb Company, Pfizer Inc; 2019.
17. Pradaxa (dabigatran). Ridgefield (CT): Boehringer Ingelheim Pharmaceuticals Inc; 2018.
18. Savaysa (edoxaban). Tokyo: Daiichi Sankyo Co.; 2019.
19. Steffel J, Verhamme P, Potpara TS, et al. The 2018 European Heart Rhythm Association Practical Guide on the use of non-vitamin K antagonist oral anticoagulants in patients with atrial fibrillation. Eur Heart J 2018;39(16):1330–93.

20. Padrini R. Clinical pharmacokinetics and pharmacodynamics of direct oral anti-coagulants in patients with renal failure. Eur J Drug Metab Pharmacokinet 2019;44(1):1–12.

21. Spyropoulos AC, Al-Badri A, Sherwood MW, et al. Periprocedural management of patients receiving a vitamin K antagonist or a direct oral anticoagulant requiring an elective procedure or surgery. J Thromb Haemost 2016;14(5):875–85.

22. Healey JS, Eikelboom J, Douketis J, et al. Periprocedural bleeding and thrombo-embolic events with dabigatran compared with warfarin: results from the Ran-domized Evaluation of Long-Term Anticoagulation Therapy (RE-LY) randomized trial. Circulation 2012;126(3):343–8.

23. Sherwood MW, Douketis JD, Patel MR, et al. Outcomes of temporary interruption of rivaroxaban compared with warfarin in patients with nonvalvular atrial fibrilla-tion: results from the rivaroxaban once daily, oral, direct factor Xa inhibition compared with vitamin K antagonism for prevention of stroke and embolism trial in atrial fibrillation (ROCKET AF). Circulation 2014;129(18):1850–9.

24. Garcia D, Alexander JH, Wallentin L, et al. Management and clinical outcomes in patients treated with apixaban vs warfarin undergoing procedures. Blood 2014; 124(25):3692–8.

25. Douketis JD, Murphy SA, Antman EM, et al. Peri-operative adverse outcomes in patients with atrial fibrillation taking warfarin or edoxaban: analysis of the ENGAGE AF-TIMI 48 trial. Thromb Haemost 2018;118(6):1001–8.

26. Granger CB, Alexander JH, McMurray JJ, et al. Apixaban versus warfarin in pa-tients with atrial fibrillation. N Engl J Med 2011;365(11):981–92.

27. Investigators RAS. Rivaroxaban-once daily, oral, direct factor Xa inhibition compared with vitamin K antagonism for prevention of stroke and Embolism Trial in Atrial Fibrillation: rationale and design of the ROCKET AF study. Am Heart J 2010;159(3):340–7.e1.

28. Giugliano RP, Ruff CT, Braunwald E, et al. Edoxaban versus warfarin in patients with atrial fibrillation. N Engl J Med 2013;369(22):2093–104.

29. Ezekowitz MD, Connolly S, Parekh A, et al. Rationale and design of RE-LY: ran-domized evaluation of long-term anticoagulant therapy, warfarin, compared with dabigatran. Am Heart J 2009;157(5):805–10, 810.e1-2.

30. Connolly SJ, Ezekowitz MD, Yusuf S, et al. Dabigatran versus warfarin in patients with atrial fibrillation. N Engl J Med 2009;361(12):1139–51.

31. Shaw JR, Woodfine JD, Douketis J, et al. Perioperative interruption of direct oral anticoagulants in patients with atrial fibrillation: a systematic review and meta-analysis. Res Pract Thromb Haemost 2018;2(2):282–90.

32. Patel MR, Mahaffey KW, Garg J, et al. Rivaroxaban versus warfarin in nonvalvular atrial fibrillation. N Engl J Med 2011;365(10):883–91.

33. Douxfils J, Lessire S, Dincq AS, et al. Estimation of dabigatran plasma concentra-tions in the perioperative setting. An ex vivo study using dedicated coagulation assays. Thromb Haemost 2015;113(4):862–9.

34. Douxfils J, Dogné JM, Mullier F, et al. Comparison of calibrated dilute thrombin time and aPTT tests with LC-MS/MS for the therapeutic monitoring of patients treated with dabigatran etexilate. Thromb Haemost 2013;110(3):543–9.

35. Douxfils J, Ageno W, Samama CM, et al. Laboratory testing in patients treated with direct oral anticoagulants: a practical guide for clinicians. J Thromb Haemost 2018;16(2):209–19.

36. Gosselin R, Grant RP, Adcock DM. Comparison of the effect of the anti-Xa direct oral anticoagulants apixaban, edoxaban, and rivaroxaban on coagulation as-says. Int J Lab Hematol 2016;38(5):505–13.

37. Tripodi A. To measure or not to measure direct oral anticoagulants before surgery or invasive procedures. J Thromb Haemost 2016;14(7):1325–7.
38. Spyropoulos AC, Al-Badri A, Sherwood MW, et al. To measure or not to measure direct oral anticoagulants before surgery or invasive procedures: comment. J Thromb Haemost 2016;14(12):2556–9.
39. Godier A, Martin AC, Leblanc I, et al. Peri-procedural management of dabigatran and rivaroxaban: duration of anticoagulant discontinuation and drug concentrations. Thromb Res 2015;136(4):763–8.
40. Pernod G, Albaladejo P, Godier A, et al. Management of major bleeding complications and emergency surgery in patients on long-term treatment with direct oral anticoagulants, thrombin or factor-Xa inhibitors: proposals of the working group on perioperative haemostasis (GIHP) - March 2013. Arch Cardiovasc Dis 2013; 106(6–7):382–93.
41. Godier A, Dincq AS, Martin AC, et al. Predictors of pre-procedural concentrations of direct oral anticoagulants: a prospective multicentre study. Eur Heart J 2017; 38(31):2431–9.
42. Douketis JD, Spyropoulos AC, Duncan J, et al. Perioperative management of patients with atrial fibrillation receiving a direct oral anticoagulant. JAMA Intern Med 2019. https://doi.org/10.1001/jamainternmed.2019.2431.
43. Schulman S, Carrier M, Lee AY, et al. Perioperative management of dabigatran: a prospective cohort study. Circulation 2015;132(3):167–73.
44. Beyer-Westendorf J, Gelbricht V, Förster K, et al. Peri-interventional management of novel oral anticoagulants in daily care: results from the prospective Dresden NOAC registry. Eur Heart J 2014;35(28):1888–96.
45. Horlocker TT, Vandermeuelen E, Kopp SL, et al. Regional anesthesia in the patient receiving antithrombotic or thrombolytic therapy: American Society of Regional Anesthesia and pain medicine evidence-based guidelines (fourth edition). Reg Anesth Pain Med 2018;43(3):263–309.
46. Woods K, Douketis JD, Kathirgamanathan K, et al. Low-dose oral vitamin K to normalize the international normalized ratio prior to surgery in patients who require temporary interruption of warfarin. J Thromb Thrombolysis 2007; 24(2):93–7.
47. Douketis J, Wang J, Cuddy K, et al. The safety of co-administered continuous epidural analgesia and low-molecular-weight heparin after major orthopedic surgery: assessment of a standardized patient management protocol. Thromb Haemost 2006;96(3):387–9.
48. Skeith L, Taylor J, Lazo-Langner A, et al. Conservative perioperative anticoagulation management in patients with chronic venous thromboembolic disease: a cohort study. J Thromb Haemost 2012;10(11):2298–304.
49. Shaw J, de Wit C, Le Gal G, et al. Thrombotic and bleeding outcomes following perioperative interruption of direct oral anticoagulants in patients with venous thromboembolic disease. J Thromb Haemost 2017;15(5):925–30.
50. Clark NP, Witt DM, Davies LE, et al. Bleeding, recurrent venous thromboembolism, and mortality risks during warfarin interruption for invasive procedures. JAMA Intern Med 2015;175(7):1163–8.
51. Baron TH, Kamath PS, McBane RD. Management of antithrombotic therapy in patients undergoing invasive procedures. N Engl J Med 2013;368(22): 2113–24.
52. Spyropoulos AC, Brohi K, Caprini J, et al. Scientific and standardization committee communication: guidance document on the periprocedural management of patients on chronic oral anticoagulant therapy: recommendations for

standardized reporting of procedural/surgical bleed risk and patient-specific thromboembolic risk. J Thromb Haemost 2019;17(11):1966–72.

53. Birnie DH, Healey JS, Wells GA, et al. Pacemaker or defibrillator surgery without interruption of anticoagulation. N Engl J Med 2013;368(22):2084–93.

54. Birnie DH, Healey JS, Wells GA, et al. Continued vs. interrupted direct oral anti-coagulants at the time of device surgery, in patients with moderate to high risk of arterial thrombo-embolic events (BRUISE CONTROL-2). Eur Heart J 2018;39(44):3973–9.

55. Di Biase L, Burkhardt JD, Santangeli P, et al. Periprocedural stroke and bleeding complications in patients undergoing catheter ablation of atrial fibrilla-tion with different anticoagulation management: results from the Role of Couma-din in Preventing Thromboembolism in Atrial Fibrillation (AF) Patients Undergoing Catheter Ablation (COMPARE) randomized trial. Circulation 2014;129(25):2638–44.

56. Jamula E, Douketis JD, Schulman S. Perioperative anticoagulation in patients having implantation of a cardiac pacemaker or defibrillator: a systematic review and practical management guide. J Thromb Haemost 2008;6(10):1615–21.

57. Jamula E, Lloyd NS, Schwalm JD, et al. Safety of uninterrupted anticoagulation in patients requiring elective coronary angiography with or without percutaneous coronary intervention: a systematic review and metaanalysis. Chest 2010;138(4):840–7.

58. Engelen ET, Schutgens RE, Mauser-Bunschoten EP, et al. Antifibrinolytic therapy for preventing oral bleeding in people on anticoagulants undergoing minor oral surgery or dental extractions. Cochrane Database Syst Rev 2018;(7):CD012293.

59. Patel JP, Woolcombe SA, Patel RK, et al. Managing direct oral anticoagulants in patients undergoing dentoalveolar surgery. Br Dent J 2017;222(4):245–9.

60. Kaplovitch E, Dounaevskaia V. Treatment in the dental practice of the patient receiving anticoagulation therapy. J Am Dent Assoc 2019;150(7):602–8.

61. Billingsley EM, Maloney ME. Intraoperative and postoperative bleeding prob-lems in patients taking warfarin, aspirin, and nonsteroidal antiinflammatory agents. A prospective study. Dermatol Surg 1997;23(5):381–3 [discussion: 384–5].

62. Kargi E, Babuccu O, Hosnuter M, et al. Complications of minor cutaneous sur-gery in patients under anticoagulant treatment. Aesthetic Plast Surg 2002;26(6):483–5.

63. Syed S, Adams BB, Liao W, et al. A prospective assessment of bleeding and in-ternational normalized ratio in warfarin-anticoagulated patients having cutaneous surgery. J Am Acad Dermatol 2004;51(6):955–7.

64. Jamula E, Anderson J, Douketis JD. Safety of continuing warfarin therapy during cataract surgery: a systematic review and meta-analysis. Thromb Res 2009;124(3):292–9.

65. Veitch AM, Vanbiervliet G, Gershlick AH, et al. Endoscopy in patients on anti-platelet or anticoagulant therapy, including direct oral anticoagulants: British So-ciety of Gastroenterology (BSG) and European Society of Gastrointestinal Endoscopy (ESGE) guidelines. Endoscopy 2016;48(4):c1.

66. Friedland S, Sedehi D, Soetikno R. Colonoscopic polypectomy in anticoagulated patients. World J Gastroenterol 2009;15(16):1973–6.

67. Horiuchi A, Nakayama Y, Kajiyama M, et al. Removal of small colorectal polyps in anticoagulated patients: a prospective randomized comparison of cold snare and conventional polypectomy. Gastrointest Endosc 2014;79(2):417–23.

Teamwork Essentials for Hospitalists

Kevin J. O'Leary, MD, MS[a],*, Krystal Hanrahan, MS, MSPH, RN, CMSRN[b],
Rachel M. Cyrus, MD[a]

KEYWORDS

- Teamwork • Interprofessional practice • Patient safety • Clinical microsystems

KEY POINTS

- Teamwork is essential for safe, effective, patient-centered care.
- Hospital settings pose important challenges to teamwork, especially in the care of general medical patients.
- Measurement of teamwork is critical to understand baseline performance and determine whether interventions are successful.
- A multifaceted approach is best, using a combination of complementary interventions that redesign systems of care.

IMPORTANCE OF TEAMWORK

Teamwork is essential to providing safe, effective, and patient-centered care. Teamwork is especially important in hospital settings, where patients with acute medical conditions undergo multiple tests and receive complex treatments.[1] Health care professionals caring for hospitalized patients spend approximately a quarter of their time on teamwork-related activities.[2,3] A large body of research has shown an association between teamwork and patient safety, with communication failure frequently identified as a contributing factor in adverse events.[4,5] Observational studies have further shown an association between teamwork culture and mortality.[6,7] Teamwork influences the health of an organization as well, with observational research showing that hospitals with higher ratings of teamwork culture have higher patient satisfaction and lower nurse resignation rates.[8,9]

[a] Division of Hospital Medicine, Northwestern University Feinberg School of Medicine, 211 East Ontario Street, 7th Floor, Chicago, IL 60611, USA; [b] Nursing Development, Magnet Program Manager, Northwestern Memorial Hospital, 251 East Huron Street, 4th Floor, Chicago, IL 60611, USA
* Corresponding author.
E-mail address: keoleary@nm.org
Twitter: @kevinjolearymd (K.J.O.); @rachelcyrus4 (R.M.C.)

Med Clin N Am 104 (2020) 727–737
https://doi.org/10.1016/j.mcna.2020.03.001
0025-7125/20/© 2020 Elsevier Inc. All rights reserved.

CHALLENGES TO TEAMWORK IN HOSPITAL MEDICINE

Several challenges impede teamwork in hospital settings. Health care teams are large and team membership changes frequently because of the need to provide care 24 hours a day. Team member workflow is seldom aligned to allow team members to be in the same place at the same time. Physicians often care for patients on multiple units and floors, whereas nurses and other team members are typically unit based.[10] Research has shown[11–13] that team size, instability, and geographic dispersion of membership serve as important barriers to improving teamwork.[11,14] As a result of these barriers, nurses and physicians do not communicate consistently and often disagree on the daily plan of care for their patients.[10,15] When communication does occur, health care professionals tend to overestimate how well their messages are understood by other team members.[16,17]

The traditionally steep hierarchy within medicine may also serve as a challenge to teamwork. Studies reveal widely discrepant views on the quality of collaboration between health care professionals.[18–20] Although physicians generally give high ratings to the quality of collaboration with nurses, nurses consistently rate the quality of collaboration with physicians as poor. Similarly, specialist physicians rate collaboration with hospitalists higher than hospitalists rate collaboration with specalists.[20] Effective teams in other high-risk industries, such as aviation, strive to flatten hierarchy so that team members feel comfortable raising concerns and engaging in open and respectful communication.[21]

Although working in an interprofessional team is common and crucial, training is still often completed in profession-specific silos and does not necessarily incorporate teamwork training. This approach leads to decreased understanding of others' roles, responsibilities, and priorities.[22–24] In addition, communication technology has traditionally lagged in health care compared with other industries, in part because of privacy concerns. For example, pagers remain the technology most commonly used by hospital-based clinicians and only a minority of health systems have yet to implement secure mobile messaging applications.[25]

TEAMWORK CONSTRUCTS AND FRAMEWORKS

A team is defined as 2 or more individuals with specified roles interacting adaptively, interdependently, and dynamically toward a shared and common goal.[12] Salas and colleagues[12] developed a useful theoretic framework for teamwork, based on their studies of teams in the military, aviation, and health care. In their framework, teamwork consists of 5 core components: team leadership, mutual performance monitoring, backup behavior, adaptability, and team orientation (**Table 1**). These components are supported by 3 coordinating mechanisms: shared mental model, closed-loop communication, and mutual trust. Related to mutual trust, psychological safety has been identified as essential to open communication.[26] Psychological safety exists when people are able to show and use themselves without fear of negative consequences to self-image, status, or career.[27]

Nelson and colleagues[28] described clinical microsystems, representing another useful framework for identifying solutions to teamwork in health care settings. A clinical microsystem is defined as the small group of people who work together in a defined setting on a regular basis to provide care.[28,29] Effective clinical microsystems have clinical aims, linked processes, a shared information environment, and measure performance outcomes. Clinical microsystems evolve over time, coexist with other microsystems, and are typically embedded in larger systems. High-value organizations deliberately design clinical microsystems to optimize their performance.[29,30] Research has identified 5 overarching characteristics associated with successful

Table 1
Teamwork components and coordinating mechanisms

Teamwork	Definition	Behavioral Examples
Component		
Team leadership	The leader directs and coordinates team members' activities	• Facilitate team problem solving • Provide performance expectations • Clarify team member roles • Assist in conflict resolution
Mutual performance monitoring	Team members are able to monitor one another's performance	• Identify mistakes and lapses in other team member actions • Provide feedback to fellow team members to facilitate self-correction
Backup behavior	Team members anticipate and respond to one another's needs	• Recognize workload distribution problem • Shift work responsibilities to underused members
Adaptability	The team adjusts strategies based on new information	• Identify cues that change has occurred and develop plan to deal with changes • Remain vigilant to change in internal and external environment
Team orientation	Team members prioritize team goals more than individual goals	• Take into account alternate solutions by teammates • Increased task involvement, information sharing, and participatory goal setting
Coordinating Mechanism		
Shared mental model	An organizing knowledge of the task of the team and how members will interact to achieve their goal	• Anticipate and predict each other's needs • Identify changes in team, task, or teammates
Closed-loop communication	Acknowledgments and confirmation of information received	• Follow up with team members to ensure message received • Acknowledge that message was received • Clarify information received
Mutual trust	Shared belief that team members will perform their roles	• Share information • Willingly admit mistakes and accept feedback

Adapted from Baker DP, Salas E, King H, et al. The role of teamwork in the professional education of physicians: current status and assessment recommendations. Jt Comm J Qual Patient Saf 2005;31(4):185-202; with permission.

microsystems: local leadership, focus on the needs of staff, emphasis on the needs of patients, attention to performance, and a rich information environment (**Fig. 1**). As mentioned earlier, medical services have challenges in each of these 5 areas (**Table 2**).

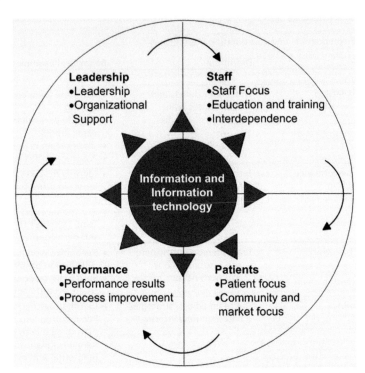

Fig. 1. The 5 characteristics of successful microsystems. (*From* Nelson EC, Batalden PB, Godfrey MM, et al. Value by design: developing clinical microsystems to achieve organizational excellence, 2nd edition. San Francisco: Jossey-Bass; 2011; with permission.)

MEASUREMENT OF TEAMWORK

Teamwork measurement is essential to understanding baseline performance and whether interventions have improved performance. Approaches to teamwork assessment include peer assessment, direct observation, and surveys of teamwork climate or culture. Peer assessment includes the use of 360° evaluations or multisource feedback, and provides evaluation of individual performance. Direct observation attempts to identify behaviors of individuals or teams that are consistent with optimal teamwork. Direct observation can be used in simulated or real-world settings, but a prerequisite is that 1 or more team members has to be in the same place at the same time to observe specific behaviors. Several tools for direct observation have been created and tested.[31] Typically, observers need training to ensure that they can reliably assess teamwork behaviors represented in the tool. An important advantage of direct observation and the use of a teamwork assessment tool is that it allows for provision of feedback to individuals to improve teamwork behaviors. Surveys of team climate or culture can also be used and have the advantage of feasibly obtaining data from a large number of individuals. Several survey instruments have been developed and tested.[32,33] An important limitation of teamwork surveys is that they do not identify problematic teamwork behaviors or allow for the provision of feedback.

INTERVENTIONS TO IMPROVE TEAMWORK IN HOSPITAL MEDICINE

Several interventions have been used to improve teamwork in hospital medicine. In general, these interventions attempt to improve professionals' teamwork skills or address the structural challenges that impede teamwork.

Table 2
Challenges on medical services by microsystem domain

Domains	Challenges
Local leadership	• Nursing and physician leaders often operate in silos • Physician leadership at the unit level may not exist • Formal training of unit leaders is often lacking
Focus on needs of staff	• Dispersion of physicians limits their connection to any particular unit • Team members inconsistently given orientation to units/services • Team member roles and expectations not defined
Emphasis on needs of patients	• Patients have poor comprehension of plan of care • Limited opportunities exist for patients and families to partner in care
Attention to performance	• Performance data often unavailable at the unit level • Limited data to prompt changes during patients' hospitalizations
Rich information environment	• Few opportunities for team members to share information and collaborate on better decisions • Technology not leveraged to identify opportunities to improve care

From O'Leary KJ, Johnson JK, Manojlovich M, et al. Redesigning systems to improve teamwork and quality for hospitalized patients (RESET): study protocol evaluating the effect of mentored implementation to redesign clinical microsystems. BMC Health Serv Res 2019;19(1):293; with permission.

Teamwork Training

Formal teamwork training programs have been implemented in several clinical environments, including the emergency department, operating room, labor and delivery suites, and intensive care units.[34–37] The evidence for the effectiveness of these teamwork training programs is mixed. Although the literature supports an association with increased knowledge of teamwork principles, attitudes about the importance of teamwork, and overall safety climate, few studies have evaluated patient outcomes.[13,38] Most studies on teamwork training have been conducted in settings where team members are typically in the same place at the same time. Sehgal and colleagues[39] studied teamwork training in the general medical hospital medicine setting and found that a multifaceted teamwork training program improved health care professional safety knowledge and attitudes and patient perceptions of teamwork and communication [Auerbach AA, Sehgal NL, Blegen MA, et al. Effects of a multicenter teamwork and communication program on patient outcomes: results from the Triad for Optimal Patient Safety (TOPS) project, under review].[40,41]

Localization of Physicians

Studies have shown that localizing physicians to specific units increases the frequency with which nurses and physicians discuss their patients' plans of care and reduces the number of pages received by physicians, presumably because of greater face-to-face communication.[42–45] Localization may also improve relationships and trust between physicians and nurses.

Unit Nurse-Physician Coleadership

Unit nurse-physician coleadership is a collaborative model in which a nurse manager and physician medical director share responsibility for quality on their unit.[46–49]

Although not rigorously evaluated, the model has been associated with reductions in central line–associated blood stream infections, catheter-associated urinary tract infections, and pressure ulcers.[50] An additional benefit of the unit coleadership model is the ability to set the stage for team collaboration. Working together, unit medical directors and nurse managers can articulate the roles, knowledge, and skills of the interprofessional team to establish a solid understanding of professional identity that is necessary for collaborative practice.[51] As unit coleaders, they help to sustain this culture of collaboration through team orientation as team membership changes.

Interprofessional Rounds

Several systematic reviews have evaluated the impact of interprofessional rounds in medical settings and found evidence to support improvements in staff satisfaction, but an inconsistent effect on length of stay.[52–54] Although the evidence suggests improvements in patient safety, few studies have evaluated the effect of interprofessional rounds on adverse events.[52,53] An important development is the use of interprofessional rounds at the bedside (also called patient and family–centered rounds) to better inform and engage patients.[55–58] A recent systematic review found that bedside rounds were associated with a small, statistically significant improvement in patient experience but no improvement in patient knowledge.[59]

BUNDLED INTERVENTIONS TO REDESIGN SYSTEMS OF CARE

Importantly, many hospitals have implemented and assessed the effect of a single intervention (eg, physician localization without unit-based nurse-physician coleadership or interprofessional rounds).[60] These interventions are better conceptualized as complementary and mutually reinforcing components of a redesigned clinical microsystem and should be implemented and evaluated as such. Although more research is needed, early research suggests that patient outcomes are improved with this approach. For example, Stein and colleagues[61] implemented an accountable care unit model, consisting of unit-based teams, unit-level nurse and physician coleadership, structured interprofessional bedside rounds, and unit-level performance reporting, on a medical unit at Emory University Hospital. Although not rigorously assessed, the interventions seemed to reduce length of stay and mortality. Kara and colleagues[62] implemented a similar model, the accountable care team model, including geographic cohorting of patients and clinicians, interprofessional bedside rounds, and monthly review of unit-level data, on 11 units at Indiana University Health Methodist Hospital. The degree to which units implemented components of the intervention was associated with improved length of stay and costs, but not patient satisfaction scores. O'Leary and colleagues[63–65] have sequentially implemented similar interventions, including localization of physicians, unit nurse-physician coleadership, structured interdisciplinary rounds, and unit-level performance reports, at Northwestern Memorial Hospital. These interventions were associated with improvements in teamwork climate and a reduction in adverse events.

More recently, a team of investigators partnered with the Society of Hospital Medicine and the American Nurses Association on the Redesigning Systems to Improve Teamwork and Quality for Hospitalized Patients (RESET) project. In this Agency for Healthcare Research and Quality–funded project, 4 hospitals receive mentorship and support as they implement the advanced and integrated microsystems (AIMS) interventions. The AIMS model includes 5 interventions and was closely modeled on prior studies (**Table 3**).[61,62,66] The RESET study will evaluate the effect of the AIMS

Table 3
Advanced and integrated microsystems interventions, supporting processes and tools

Components	Descriptions	Supporting Processes and Tools
Unit-based physician teams	Localization of physicians to a minimal number of units on which they provide patient care	• Projecting expected patient volume • Engaging stakeholders to redesign admission processes • Monitoring progress and making adjustments
Unit nurse-physician coleadership	Collaborative model in which a nurse leader and physician leader are jointly responsible for quality improvement on their unit	• Coleader selection and training • Coleader job descriptions and activities • Establishing unit norms and values • Coleader integration into mesosystem activities
Enhanced interprofessional rounds	Interprofessional rounds, redesigned with input from frontline professionals to optimize collaboration and patient engagement	• Redesign work groups; determine timing, format, duration, and location • Discussions facilitated by unit coleaders • Roles/expectations of attendees defined • Structured tools to support closed-loop communication
Unit-level performance reports	Performance reports designed to give unit leaders and frontline professionals relevant, interpretable, actionable data	• Monthly unit-level reports aligned with organizational priorities • Daily reports to identify opportunities to improve care • Just-in-time reports to identify opportunities to improve care • Teamwork climate survey reports
Patient engagement activities	Methods to continually inform and engage patients and families as partners in care	• Use of whiteboards to define goals and the daily care plan • Patient experience rounds by unit coleaders • Conducting interprofessional rounds and nurse shift reports at bedside

From O'Leary KJ, Johnson JK, Manojlovich M, et al. Redesigning systems to improve teamwork and quality for hospitalized patients (RESET): study protocol evaluating the effect of mentored implementation to redesign clinical microsystems. BMC Health Serv Res 2019;19(1):293; with permission.

interventions on patient outcomes and factors associated with successful implementation.

SUMMARY

Teamwork is essential to providing high-quality patient care. Hospital settings pose important challenges to teamwork. Measurement is key to understanding baseline performance and assessing whether teamwork is improving. The authors recommend a multifaceted approach, using a combination of complementary interventions, with the ultimate goal of translating improved teamwork into improved patient outcomes.

DISCLOSURE

Dr. O'Leary and Ms. Hanrahan received support from a grant from the Agency for Healthcare Research and Quality (AHRQ). R18 HS25649. AHRQ played no role in writing this review or the decision to submit the review for publication.

REFERENCES

1. Schmutz JB, Meier LL, Manser T. How effective is teamwork really? The relationship between teamwork and performance in healthcare teams: a systematic review and meta-analysis. BMJ Open 2019;9(9):e028280.
2. Keohane CA, Bane AD, Featherstone E, et al. Quantifying nursing workflow in medication administration. J Nurs Adm 2008;38(1):19–26.
3. Tipping MD, Forth VE, O'Leary KJ, et al. Where did the day go?–a time-motion study of hospitalists. J Hosp Med 2010;5(6):323–8.
4. Patient Safety. Sentinel Event Statistics Released for 2014. The Joint Commission: The Joint Commission; April 29, 2015 2015. Available at: https://www.jointcommission.org/-/media/deprecated-unorganized/imported-assets/tjc/system-folders/joint-commission-online/jconline_april_29_15pdf.pdf?db=web&hash=DEFFBC41623A360F1C1428A5E9602773.
5. Sutcliffe KM, Lewton E, Rosenthal MM. Communication failures: an insidious contributor to medical mishaps. Acad Med 2004;79(2):186–94.
6. Baggs JG, Schmitt MH, Mushlin AI, et al. Association between nurse-physician collaboration and patient outcomes in three intensive care units. Crit Care Med 1999;27(9):1991–8.
7. Wheelan SA, Burchill CN, Tilin F. The link between teamwork and patients' outcomes in intensive care units. Am J Crit Care 2003;12(6):527–34.
8. Meterko M, Mohr DC, Young GJ. Teamwork culture and patient satisfaction in hospitals. Med Care 2004;42(5):492–8.
9. Mohr DC, Burgess JF Jr, Young GJ. The influence of teamwork culture on physician and nurse resignation rates in hospitals. Health Serv Manag Res 2008;21(1):23–31.
10. O'Leary KJ, Thompson JA, Landler MP, et al. Patterns of nurse-physician communication and agreement on the plan of care. Qual Saf Health Care 2010;19(3):195–9.
11. Salas E, DiazGranados D, Klein C, et al. Does team training improve team performance? A meta-analysis. Hum Factors 2008;50(6):903–33.
12. Salas E, Sims DE, Burke CS. Is there a "big five" in teamwork? Small Group Res 2005;36:555–99.

13. Salas E, Wilson KA, Burke CS, et al. Does crew resource management training work? An update, an extension, and some critical needs. Hum Factors 2006; 48(2):392–412.

14. Lemieux-Charles L, McGuire WL. What do we know about health care team effectiveness? A review of the literature. Med Care Res Rev 2006;63(3):263–300.

15. Evanoff B, Potter P, Wolf L, et al. Advances in Patient safety. Can we talk? Priorities for patient care differed among health care providers. In: Henriksen K, Battles JB, Marks ES, et al, editors. Advances in patient safety: from research to implementation (volume 1: research findings). Rockville (MD): Agency for Healthcare Research and Quality (US); 2005. p. 5–14.

16. Chang VY, Arora VM, Lev-Ari S, et al. Interns overestimate the effectiveness of their hand-off communication. Pediatrics 2010;125(3):491–6.

17. Keysar B, Henly AS. Speakers' overestimation of their effectiveness. Psychol Sci 2002;13(3):207–12.

18. Makary MA, Sexton JB, Freischlag JA, et al. Operating room teamwork among physicians and nurses: teamwork in the eye of the beholder. J Am Coll Surg 2006;202(5):746–52.

19. Thomas EJ, Sexton JB, Helmreich RL. Discrepant attitudes about teamwork among critical care nurses and physicians. Crit Care Med 2003;31(3):956–9.

20. O'Leary KJ, Ritter CD, Wheeler H, et al. Teamwork on inpatient medical units: assessing attitudes and barriers. Qual Saf Health Care 2010;19(2):117–21.

21. Sexton JB, Thomas EJ, Helmreich RL. Error, stress, and teamwork in medicine and aviation: cross sectional surveys. BMJ 2000;320(7237):745–9.

22. Watson K, Mainwaring C, Moran A, et al. Interprofessional bedside teaching: setting up a novel teaching programme. Br J Hosp Med (Lond) 2017;78(12): 716–8.

23. Weller J, Boyd M, Cumin D. Teams, tribes and patient safety: overcoming barriers to effective teamwork in healthcare. Postgrad Med J 2014;90(1061):149–54.

24. Pullon S. Competence, respect and trust: key features of successful interprofessional nurse-doctor relationships. J interprofessional Care 2008;22(2):133–47.

25. O'Leary KJ, Liebovitz DM, Wu RC, et al. Hospital-based clinicians' use of technology for patient care-related communication: a national survey. J Hosp Med 2017; 12(7):530–5.

26. Edmondson AC. Managing the risk of learning: psychological safety in work teams. In: West MA, Tjosvold D, Smith KG, editors. International handbook of organizational teamwork and cooperative working. New York: Wiley; 2003. p. 255–75.

27. Kahn WA. Psychological conditions of personal engagement and disengagement at work. Acad Managment J 1990;33(4):692–724.

28. Nelson EC, Batalden PB, Huber TP, et al. Microsystems in health care: Part 1. Learning from high-performing front-line clinical units. The Joint Comm J Qual improvement 2002;28(9):472–93.

29. Nelson EC, Batalden PB, Godfrey MM, et al. Value by design: developing clinical microsystems to achieve organizational excellence. 2nd edition. San Francisco (CA): Jossey-Bass; 2011.

30. Bohmer RM. The four habits of high-value health care organizations. New Engl J Med 2011;365(22):2045–7.

31. Higham H, Greig PR, Rutherford J, et al. Observer-based tools for non-technical skills assessment in simulated and real clinical environments in healthcare: a systematic review. BMJ Qual Saf 2019;28(8):672–86.

32. Havyer RD, Wingo MT, Comfere NI, et al. Teamwork assessment in internal medicine: a systematic review of validity evidence and outcomes. J Gen Intern Med 2014;29(6):894–910.

33. Valentine MA, Nembhard IM, Edmondson AC. Measuring teamwork in health care settings: a review of survey instruments. Med Care 2015;53(4):e16–30.

34. Awad SS, Fagan SP, Bellows C, et al. Bridging the communication gap in the operating room with medical team training. Am J Surg 2005;190(5):770–4.

35. Morey JC, Simon R, Jay GD, et al. Error reduction and performance improvement in the emergency department through formal teamwork training: evaluation results of the MedTeams project. Health Serv Res 2002;37(6):1553–81.

36. Nielsen PE, Goldman MB, Mann S, et al. Effects of teamwork training on adverse outcomes and process of care in labor and delivery: a randomized controlled trial. Obstet Gynecol 2007;109(1):48–55.

37. Sherwood G, Thomas E, Bennett DS, et al. A teamwork model to promote patient safety in critical care. Crit Care Nurs Clin North Am 2002;14(4):333–40.

38. Hughes AM, Gregory ME, Joseph DL, et al. Saving lives: A meta-analysis of team training in healthcare. J Appl Psychol 2016;101(9):1266–304.

39. Sehgal NL, Fox M, Vidyarthi AR, et al. A multidisciplinary teamwork training program: the Triad for Optimal Patient Safety (TOPS) experience. J Gen Intern Med 2008;23(12):2053–7.

40. Blegen MA, Sehgal NL, Alldredge BK, et al. Improving safety culture on adult medical units through multidisciplinary teamwork and communication interventions: the TOPS Project. Qual Saf Health Care 2010;19(4):346–50.

41. Auerbach AD, Sehgal NL, Blegen MA. Effects of a multicentre teamwork and communication programme on patient outcomes: results from the Triad for Optimal Patient Safety (TOPS) project. BMJ Qual Saf 2012;21(2):118–26.

42. Fanucchi L, Unterbrink M, Logio LS. (Re)turning the pages of residency: the impact of localizing resident physicians to hospital units on paging frequency. J Hosp Med 2014;9(2):120–2.

43. Singh S, Tarima S, Rana V, et al. Impact of localizing general medical teams to a single nursing unit. J Hosp Med 2012;7(7):551–6.

44. Mueller SK, Schnipper JL, Giannelli K, et al. Impact of regionalized care on concordance of plan and preventable adverse events on general medicine services. J Hosp Med 2016;11(9):620–7.

45. O'Leary KJ, Wayne DB, Landler MP, et al. Impact of localizing physicians to hospital units on nurse-physician communication and agreement on the plan of care. J Gen Intern Med 2009;24(11):1223–7.

46. Clark RC, Greenawald M. Nurse-physician leadership: insights into interprofessional collaboration. J Nurs Adm 2013;43(12):653–9.

47. Kim CS, Calarco M, Jacobs T, et al. Leadership at the front line: a clinical partnership model on general care inpatient units. Am J Med Qual 2012;27(2):106–11.

48. Kim CS, King E, Stein J, et al. Unit-based interprofessional leadership models in six US hospitals. J Hosp Med 2014;9(8):545–50.

49. Rich V, Brennan PJ, Riley-Wasserman E, et al. Unit clinical leadership model: a successful partnership between front-line clinicians, quality, and senior leaders. Boston, MA: Institute for Healthcare Improvement (IHI) National Forum on Quality Improvement in Health Care; 2009. Available at: http://www.cfar.com/sites/default/files/resources/Unit_Clin_Leadership_Model.pdf.

50. Rich VL, Brennan PJ. Improvement Projects Led by Unit-Based Teams of Nurse, Physician, and Quality Leaders Reduce Infections, Lower Costs, Improve Patient Satisfaction, and Nurse–Physician Communication. 2014. Available at: https://

innovations.ahrq.gov/profiles/improvement-projects-led-unit-based-teams-nurse-physician-and-quality-leaders-reduce. Accessed April 30, 2019.
51. Orchard CA. Persistent isolationist or collaborator? The nurse's role in interprofessional collaborative practice. J Nurs Manag 2010;18(3):248–57.
52. Bhamidipati VS, Elliott DJ, Justice EM, et al. Structure and outcomes of interdisciplinary rounds in hospitalized medicine patients: A systematic review and suggested taxonomy. J Hosp Med 2016;11(7):513–23.
53. Pannick S, Davis R, Ashrafian H, et al. Effects of interdisciplinary team care interventions on general medical wards: a systematic review. JAMA Intern Med 2015; 175(8):1288–98.
54. Zwarenstein M, Goldman J, Reeves S. Interprofessional collaboration: effects of practice-based interventions on professional practice and healthcare outcomes. Cochrane Database Syst Rev 2009;(3):CD000072.
55. Dunn AS, Reyna M, Radbill B, et al. The impact of bedside interdisciplinary rounds on length of stay and complications. J Hosp Med 2017;12(3):137–42.
56. Gonzalo JD, Kuperman E, Lehman E, et al. Bedside interprofessional rounds: perceptions of benefits and barriers by internal medicine nursing staff, attending physicians, and housestaff physicians. J Hosp Med 2014;9(10):646–51.
57. Gonzalo JD, Wolpaw DR, Lehman E, et al. Patient-centered interprofessional collaborative care: factors associated with bedside interprofessional rounds. J Gen Intern Med 2014;29(7):1040–7.
58. O'Leary KJ, Killarney A, Hansen LO, et al. Effect of patient-centred bedside rounds on hospitalised patients' decision control, activation and satisfaction with care. BMJ Qual Saf 2016;25(12):921–8.
59. Ratelle JT, Sawatsky AP, Kashiwagi DT, et al. Implementing bedside rounds to improve patient-centred outcomes: a systematic review. BMJ Qual Saf 2019; 28(4):317–26.
60. O'Leary KJ, Johnson JK, Manojlovich M, et al. Use of unit-based interventions to improve the quality of care for hospitalized medical patients: a national survey. Jt Comm J Qual Patient Saf 2017;43(11):573–9.
61. Stein J, Payne C, Methvin A, et al. Reorganizing a hospital ward as an accountable care unit. J Hosp Med 2015;10(1):36–40.
62. Kara A, Johnson CS, Nicley A, et al. Redesigning inpatient care: Testing the effectiveness of an accountable care team model. J Hosp Med 2015;10(12):773–9.
63. O'Leary KJ, Buck R, Fligiel HM, et al. Structured interdisciplinary rounds in a medical teaching unit: improving patient safety. Arch Intern Med 2011;171(7): 678–84.
64. O'Leary KJ, Haviley C, Slade ME, et al. Improving teamwork: impact of structured interdisciplinary rounds on a hospitalist unit. J Hosp Med 2011;6(2):88–93.
65. O'Leary KJ, Wayne DB, Haviley C, et al. Improving teamwork: impact of structured interdisciplinary rounds on a medical teaching unit. J Gen Intern Med 2010;25(8):826–32.
66. O'Leary KJ, Creden AJ, Slade ME, et al. Implementation of unit-based interventions to improve teamwork and patient safety on a medical service. Am J Med Qual 2015;30(5):409–16.

Using Bedside Rounds to Change Culture

Abigail Bryne, MD[1], Jeff Wiese, MD[*,1]

KEYWORDS

- Bedside rounds • Culture • Patient-centered care • Supervision
- Student presentations • Autonomy

KEY POINTS

- Bedside rounds provide an opportunity for the attending physician to optimize the culture of the team, and the culture of each patient encounter, aligning both toward the shared expectations and beliefs that lead to best patient care.
- Bedside rounds provide an opportunity to observe how individual members of the team interact with the patient, enabling a better assessment of learners' position on the supervision-to-autonomy spectrum.
- The attending physician's preparation before rounds is essential to enacting effective bedside rounds.
- Properly performed, the introductions set the stage for establishing the optimal choreography of the room. With the proper arrangement, the attending has a primary line of sight to the learner presenting the patient's information, which is in the same direction as a line of sight to the patient's face.
- Selectively choosing the patients for which bedside rounds will be conducted enables a higher quality of bedside rounds experience for the team and another opportunity to assess learners' ability to accurately assess the severity of illness.

INTRODUCTION

The role of the attending physician is to ensure that the resident's diagnostic and treatment plans are accurate and safe, and to teach residents about medical topics in the context of delivering care. However, the most effective attending physicians engage in deeper responsibilities: role modeling the profession, correctly assessing and affording autonomy to learners based on their abilities, and establishing a team culture that drives best decisions in the attending's absence.[1] In short, the most effective attending physicians fulfill Bloom's taxonomy by engaging in the instruction of the

Department of Internal Medicine, Tulane University, 1430 Tulane Avenue SL-15, New Orleans, LA 70115, USA
[1] Present Address: Department of Medicine; SL-50, Tulane University Health Sciences Center New Orleans, LA 70112.
* Corresponding author.
E-mail address: jwiese@tulane.edu

Med Clin N Am 104 (2020) 739–750
https://doi.org/10.1016/j.mcna.2020.02.008
0025-7125/20/© 2020 Elsevier Inc. All rights reserved.

attitudes as much as the knowledge and skills, which lead to best team-based patient-centered care.[2]

Multiple studies have extolled the value of bedside rounds. Patients who experienced bedside rounds were more likely to report more physician time spent at the bedside, more favorable perceptions of their care, and a greater sense of compassion on the part of the provider team.[3–5] Family rounds at the bedside have been shown to improve patient satisfaction pertaining to physician communication and support for family decision making.[6] A qualitative survey demonstrated that patients felt a sense of helpfulness to the team by contributing to education, learned about their medical conditions, and found it to be a welcome social encounter in an otherwise isolating hospitalization.[7] A survey of learners found that those exposed to bedside rounds had a higher preference for bedside rounds and that they believed it was important for learning clinical skills.[8]

BARRIERS TO BEDSIDE ROUNDS

However, not all studies have been equally supportive of bedside rounds. One study found that residents were less likely to believe that bedside rounds were educational.[9] A meta-analysis of studies addressing patient satisfaction and patient understanding of their disease failed to show a difference between bedside versus non-bedside rounds.[10] Although one study found a significant difference in the compassion the patient felt toward their provider team, it failed to show differences in perceived involvement, trust of the team, or satisfaction.[5]

There are many psychological barriers that create a cognitive bias against bedside rounds. There is a perception that "table rounds" are more efficient and expedient. Similarly, there is the fear that one loquacious patient will limit time for other patients, thereby compromising attending rounds. The pressure of increasing census size, patient intensity, and limited resident duty hours has amplified these concerns. There are also the fears of presenting sensitive data in front of the patient, the emotional impact of residents presenting inaccurate data in front of the patient, and the psychological discomfort to residents and students in presenting in front of the patient.

UNDERSTANDING THE DISCORDANCE IN THE EVIDENCE

The discordance might be explained by the dynamic and heterogeneous nature of the inpatient environment. Not all patient encounters might be suitable for bedside rounds, and the intensity or volume of the service might make bedside rounds less amenable. However, the discordance might also be explained by *how* bedside rounds are conducted. A survey of "experienced bedside teachers" on the benefits of bedside rounds includes learner skill development, opportunity for direct observation and feedback, role modeling, team building, improved patient care, and the culture of patient-centered care.[11] Similar to that seen with the physical examination literature, the effectiveness of bedside rounds might predicate on the skill of the attending physician in executing effective bedside rounds.[1] Strategies and tactics to optimize the benefits from the approach might mitigate the barriers that preclude effective bedside rounds.

STRATEGIES AND TACTICS TO OPTIMIZE BEDSIDE ROUNDS
The Purpose of Bedside Rounds

Effective bedside rounds begin with identifying the unique value that can be obtained at the bedside rather than at a table, and restructuring rounds to optimize these benefits. In addition to instructing the knowledge and skills of medicine that cannot be learned at the table (ie, physical examination, patient communication skills), bedside rounds offer an opportunity to instruct the attitudes of medicine. In doing so, it is an opportunity to change the team's culture: the shared roles, goals, expectations, and beliefs (**Box 1**).

Each team has its own culture, and the culture will govern the decisions made by the team when no one is watching. This is important because for a typical ward service, the attending will be directly present with the team for 15 hours per week; the decisions made by the team in the remaining hours of the 80-hour working week will be governed by the team's culture. Each patient encounter also has its own culture, predicated on how much the team and the patient have established their shared roles, goals, expectations, and beliefs of that encounter. The purpose of bedside rounds, as outlined in the strategies and tactics (see later discussion), is to own and optimize the culture of the team and the culture of each patient encounter, aligning both toward the shared expectations and beliefs that lead to best care.

An additional purpose of bedside rounds is to observe how individual members of the team interact with the patient. In this context, there are valuable "tells" to give the attending physician insight as to how much autonomy should be afforded to each individual team member. This is important because optimizing autonomy for each learner is synonymous with growth, and a powerful antidote for preventing disengagement and burnout. However, autonomy hinges on trust. Giving autonomy that is not earned is unsafe, and the attending physician needs information as to how much autonomy (trust) should be afforded to each individual learner (**Fig. 1**).

Setting Expectations

It is equally important that all members of the team are in touch with the purpose and goals of bedside rounds. The initial expectation session should include the explicit expectations that bedside rounds will occur, that not all patients will be presented via bedside rounds, that the resident team leader will be responsible for identifying the

---

Box 1
Opportunities via bedside rounds

1. Instruct the attitudes of effective care: patient-centered care and patient primacy
2. Define and optimize the culture of the team, with shared expectations and beliefs around patient-centered care
3. Define and optimize the culture of the patient encounter, aligning shared expectations and beliefs that lead to best care
4. Observe how team members interact with the patient, the strength of their bond with the patient
5. Establish the learner as the patient's doctor, thereby building the therapeutic relationship between the two
6. Incorporate the patient to ensure data collected by team members is accurate
7. Assess learner's interpersonal, communication, and patient care skills
8. Reveal to the patient how much intellectual and emotional effort team members have put into their care
9. Assist learners in finding comfort with being at the bedside
10. Assess where learners are on the supervision-to-autonomy spectrum
11. Model how to manage difficult patient encounters (errors, giving bad news)

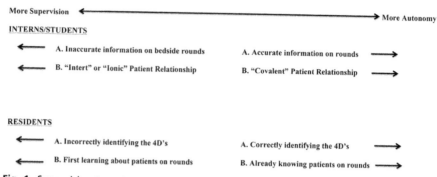

Fig. 1. Supervision-to-autonomy spectrum.

patients most amenable to bedside rounds, and that team members will be responsible for presenting at the bedside.[12] It is important that the attending establish the rationale for these expectations: bedside rounds are an opportunity to observe how team members interact with the patient, to establish bonds between the patient and team members, to ensure data collected by team members is accurate, to reveal to the patient how much effort team members have put into their care, and to establish comfort with being at the bedside.

It is useful to acknowledge that presenting in front of a patient might induce stress and fear on the part of some team members. The attending should acknowledge that finding comfort at the bedside is a natural part of transcending into the physician's role, and that the attending will be there to ensure that no one is embarrassed. The goal is that each team member learns to overcome that fear/stress, developing a new comfort with being at the bedside. Preparing for the adversity minimizes the emotional effect of the adversity.[13]

Establishing that not all patients will be presented at the bedside has 2 purposes. First, it establishes that there will be a fixed end time to rounds, and team members should plan on focusing on the experience while at the bedside, knowing that there will be a time to answer pages, place orders, and so forth at the conclusion of rounds. The second purpose is to ensure that the team leader knows of their responsibility in identifying patients who will be seen by the whole team via bedside rounds each day. A useful criterion is the 4D Criteria. Prioritization of patients for bedside rounds should be those (1) who are in *Dire* condition, (2) who have anticipated *Discharge* that day, and (3) who have active *Diagnostic* questions (eg, consults, radiographic tests).[12] Conversely, the fourth D (*Diarrhea*: those who are under contact precautions), are best seen after rounds have concluded. The attending and the primary team member responsible for seeing these patients can still see these patients together after rounds. This minimizes the number of team members in the room, optimizes infection control, and accelerates the pace of attending rounds by minimizing the time invested in gowning and gloving the entire team.

Time-Management Strategies

Optimizing time management is essential to enacting effective bedside rounds. The first strategy is to limit the number of patients who will receive bedside rounds with the entire team for that particular day. Every patient needs to be seen by the attending physician each day, but not every patient needs to be seen with the whole team each day. Attempting to see every patient at the bedside, especially with a busy service, will result in excessively long attending rounds that precludes the team enacting patient care management. Alternatively, bedside rounds for each patient will become so brief that the time at the bedside takes on the feel of a perfunctory few minutes. The lesson learned will be that the purpose of bedside rounds is nothing more than to drop in and inform the patient as to what would be changed today, a lesson antithetical to patient-centered decision making.

Establishing a fixed end time for rounds is important because it enables the team to fully engage with the experience while at the bedside. To achieve the full benefits of bedside rounds, it is important that each member of the team is mentally as well as physically present during the experience. If rounds are perceived to be perpetual, there is no impediment to immediately responding to a page or breaking away to write an order; stepping away to keep patient care moving becomes an imperative. Setting an end time to rounds allows the team to focus on the patient in front of them, knowing that there will soon be a time when rounds conclude, to write orders and return calls.

Preparation: the "Lab Spy"

Effective bedside rounds begin with knowing something about each patient before the initiation of rounds. The advantage of the electronic medical record is that it allows "spying" on each patient before the initiation of rounds. Even though there will be new information presented on rounds, reviewing notes and laboratory/radiographic studies ahead of time provides the attending a gestalt of each patient. There are 7 purposes to the lab spy, which are listed in **Box 2**.

Setting and sticking to end times for rounds predicates on the attending physician appropriately budgeting time for rounds. A larger census, or a more complex patient panel, will necessitate being more expedient on rounds, and/or choosing fewer patients with whom the attending will see with the team at the bedside. A lower census or less severe illness will afford greater latitude on rounds for extended teaching or seeing more patients with the team.

Properly performed, the attending's mental bandwidth during bedside rounds will be split between acquiring patient information/making management decisions and observing how the team interacts with the patient. If the attending physician is learning about the patient's information for the first time on attending rounds, there will be insufficient bandwidth to conduct the observations in the room necessary to make appropriate decisions regarding autonomy and supervision. An important part of the lab spy is to acquire some of the patient data ahead of rounds, thereby opening up more mental bandwidth for assessment during rounds.

The lab spy also enables the attending to identify inaccurate data in student presentations. Decisions will be made on rounds based on the data in the student

---

Box 2
Goals of the "lab spy" before rounds

1. Time manage the day

2. Open bandwidth for assessment of learners on rounds

3. Identify inaccurate data in student presentations

4. Diagnose and correct poor student presentations

5. Select teaching topics/scripts

6. Assess the resident's ability to identify "sick" versus "not sick"

7. Cardinal Rule: Supervise without Doing Their Job

presentations, and the quality of those decisions is predicated on the accuracy of the information presented. Bedside rounds augment this accuracy by allowing the patient to hear, edit, and validate what has been presented. However, having a gestalt of each patient ahead of time is another level of assurance that the data being presented on rounds are accurate.

Reviewing the chart before oral presentations on rounds enables the attending to properly diagnose and correct poor student presentations. Three of the most common causes of poor presentations are inadequate data collection, poor clinical reasoning, and nervousness in public speaking.[14] A poor oral presentation preceded by a strong admission note (ie, it has all of the relevant information, is properly organized, and has a cogent assessment and plan), is more likely to be due to poor speaking skills or nervousness. Conversely, a poor oral presentation preceded by a poor admission note is more likely to be due to poor data acquisition, organization, or clinical reasoning.

An ancillary benefit of the lab spy is to select teaching topics to be incorporated on attending rounds. The eventual goal is for the attending to develop teaching scripts for common teaching topics that require no advanced preparation.[12] However, there will invariably be diseases and conditions that are less commonly encountered, requiring some advanced preparation for instruction. Identifying these topics via the lab spy enables the attending to prepare teaching scripts on these topics in advance of attending rounds.

Given that not all patients will be seen via bedside rounds, the lab spy enables the attending to make a prerounds prediction as to which patients he or she would *expect* the resident to choose for bedside rounds. This is important in ensuring that "sick" patients are not missed on attending rounds, but it is equally important in identifying whether the resident has mastered the skill of identifying patients as "sick versus not sick," because the 4D criteria is defined by this skill. This is a valuable "tell" in assessing autonomy to be afforded to the resident. If the attending's prediction matches what the resident chooses, this is an indication that the resident should be afforded more autonomy. If the two do not match, the resident stays further to the left on the supervision to autonomy spectrum (see **Fig. 1**).

The most important part of the lab spy, however, is to ensure that the resident is being closely supervised without being aware. This enables fidelity to the attending's cardinal rule: the resident must be supervised, but the resident can never see the attending duplicating their job. The consequences of not supervising the resident's decisions are obvious. Less obvious are the consequences of oversupervising the resident to the point of doing her or his job. Although the attending physician can role-model portions of the resident's job, fully duplicating their job robs the resident of autonomy and purpose and demotivates the resident from fully completing the job.

Entry to the Room

Another strategy to optimize time management is to not round twice: rounding first in the hallway outside the patient's room, then repeating those same discussions in the patient's room. This can be accomplished by directly entering the patient's room, preceded by the question to the team, "Is there anything so super sensitive that it cannot be discussed in the room?" The nature of the question, and how it is asked, indirectly communicates to the team the answer: with very few exceptions, there is nothing so supersensitive that it cannot be discussed at the bedside in front of the patient. This is the patient's information, and he or she is entitled to hear it, despite the discomfort physicians might feel in discussing bad news.

It has become common practice for residents to wash their hands on entering a patient's room and again on leaving. It is a less common practice for *everyone* on the team to do the same, especially those who expect to not participate directly in the patient's care. The reason for this is that each team member is making an internal decision: "Is there a purpose for me to wash my hands, especially when I see no value in doing so if I am not going to touch the patient?" The attending might even be compelled by such a question, but not forcing all members to wash their hands on entry and exit of a patient's room is an opportunity missed. The act of washing hands before entering a patient's room, even if contact is not anticipated, is a moment of inconvenience; a moment of self-sacrifice when the desires of the student are subjected to a higher purpose. In short, it is a mental reminder that the patient's room is a sacred space.[15] Enforcing the standard for each member of the team is an opportunity to develop this new belief/attitude. It is easier to act your way into new beliefs then it is to believe your way into new actions, and the routine action of this self-sacrifice, albeit small, is a useful way for students to act their way into a new attitude of professionalism. Taking the time to ensure proper attire on rounds, and not having food or drinks on rounds, are similar forms of self-sacrifice that will eventually optimize the attitude of patient-first professionalism.

Introductions

One of the core elements of establishing the culture in each patient's room is establishing the "shared expectations and roles." The attending physician's entry introduction establishes the foundation for this culture. "Hello, Mr. Hamm. I hope you remember me... I am Dr. Phaedrus... the doctor that supervises your doctors." This line communicates that the role of the attending physician is not *to be* the patient's doctor, but rather *to supervise* the patient's doctor. In doing so, the attending is setting up the student/resident responsible for the patient's care to assume the role of the patient's physician.

The second level of introductions consolidates this message and further establishes the resident as the patient's primary physician. "Who here is responsible for Mr. Hamm?" The semantics of the question are important because it communicates that this "Mr. Hamm" is a person, not "a patient." In doing so, it communicates to the resident the gravity of the responsibility of assuming care for a person. These 2 introductions are designed to establish "shared expectations and roles," and are designed to establish a bond between the resident and patient that will be necessary for optimal patient care when the attending is not present.

This second level of introductions is also a potential "tell" as to how much autonomy should be afforded to the resident. If, on hearing this question, the patient appears equally curious as to who his physician might be, it is a sign that there has not been a bond established between the resident and the patient. This will necessitate tighter supervision.

Choreography

Figs. 2–4 illustrate the options for choreography in the room. In **Fig. 2**, the entire team stays at the foot of the patient's bed. The arrangement impairs the attending physician's view of the patient and the supervising resident as the student or intern is presenting the patient's information. Psychologically the team is separated from the patient, and the patient's participation in the discussion is physically impaired. Finally, the attending and the team are physically out of position to replicate and verify physical examination findings.

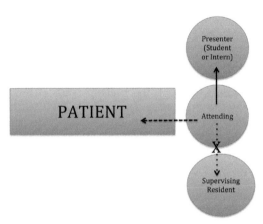

Fig. 2. Choreography of bedside rounds. The entire team stays at the foot of the patient's bed.

The choreography in **Fig. 3** moves the team closer to the patient, enabling replicating and verifying physical examination findings, but the lines of sight are still compromised and the patient remains physically detached from the discussion.

Properly performed, the introductions set the stage for establishing the optimal choreography of the room (see **Fig. 4**). After the "person responsible for Mr. Hamm" is identified, the attending physician is in a position to ask, "Thank you. Please stand over here" (the head of the patient's bed, on the patient's left side). The supervising resident is instructed to stand on the patient's left side, at the middle to the foot of the patient's bed. The attending then assumes a position at the midpoint of the patient's right side.

With this arrangement, the attending has a primary line of sight to the student/intern presenting the patient's information, which is in the same direction as a line of sight to the patient's face (see **Fig. 4**). This enables the attending to read the expressions of the patient's face as the information is presented. A furrowing of the brow suggests that the information presented might be inaccurate; a raising of the brow suggests that the patient is concerned or fearful. In either situation, the attending is in a position to pause the presentation and clarify the information or comfort the patient. The accuracy of the data being presented is a "tell" for the attending physician: consistently accurate information affords the student/intern with more autonomy, whereas a pattern of inaccurate information requires greater supervision (see **Fig. 1**).

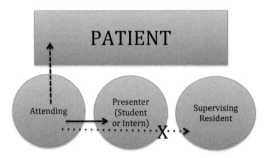

Fig. 3. Choreography of bedside rounds. The team moves closer to the patient.

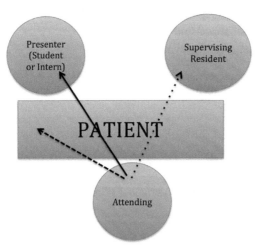

Fig. 4. Choreography of bedside rounds. Introductions set the stage for establishing the optimal choreography.

As with table rounds, the attending's primary role on bedside rounds is to augment his or her understanding of each patient's condition and ensure that the correct management plan has been established. However, unlike table rounds, the attending's role on bedside rounds has additional purposes, the first of which is identifying the nature of the student-patient "bond." There is a spectrum of this interaction, ranging from "inert" (impersonal) to "ionic" (polite, but formal) to "covalent" (personable). The "inert" relationship is characterized by a complete absence of patient-learner interaction; the presenter's presentation will be focused on the disease and not the person, frequently using impersonal pronouns (ie, "the patient says…" instead of "she says…"). There will be more patient-presenter interaction in the "ionic" relationship, but it will feel impersonal and forced, as if the intern was merely playing a role. The covalent relationship will have the feel of a true interpersonal connection, as if 2 friends were catching up. The patient is the focus of the presentation, with frequent use of personal pronouns or the patient's name. The presentation will be frequently interrupted by side-bar discussions between the presenter and the patient, as if the remainder of the team was not present.

Although the patient's personality can influence this assessment, an assessment of how individual learners interact with multiple patients can be a valuable "tell" in how much autonomy they should be afforded (see **Fig. 1**). Covalency arises from experience, comfort in talking with patients, a personal connection with patients, and frequent prior conversations in the patient's room. This portends a higher probability that the learner will identify accurate patient information, changes in the patient's condition, and patient-centered preferences in care. All of these portend safer patient care, affording an increase in resident autonomy.

The positioning of the supervising resident is also important because this individual remains in the attending physician's peripheral vision. A supervising resident who is furiously writing down the patient's information as it is being presented is a "tell" for the attending. Although he or she might have been an exceptional intern, (s)he has not fully mastered managing patients by proxy in supervising the interns/students. Accordingly, he or she will require greater supervision (see **Fig. 1**). Conversely, the resident who seems to be in sync with the student's presentation, easily providing additions or edits, has demonstrated ability to manage patients by proxy. A greater autonomy should be afforded to this resident.

The Attending's Position in the Room

The attending's physical presence in the room is equally important. Sitting or kneeling, as opposed to standing, offers additional advantages. At this lower level, the attending is physically at the elevation of the patient, decreasing psychological size[16] and further inviting the patient into the discussion. This also better aligns the lines of sight to the patient and the presenter. Sitting or kneeling, instead of standing, at a patient's bedside improves patient satisfaction, patient compliance, and provider-patient rapport.[16,17] Furthermore, patients perceive their provider as spending more time at the bedside.[18,19]

To be on the right or left side of the patient is largely a style choice, although being on the right side of the patient better enables some physical examination maneuvers (ie, feeling for the point of maximal impulse, palpating the liver).

Feedback and Out-Take

When to give feedback during attending rounds is a common dilemma. As addressed earlier, errors in historical information or management decisions should be addressed at the bedside lest the patient be confused as to the correct decision and plan. Whenever possible, it is important for the attending to neutralize the error by explaining how it was understandable to have come to that conclusion, but with greater experience the better course is an alternative course. This should be followed quickly by an affirmation that the decisions we make are often complex and difficult, and this is the reason for team-based bedside rounds: collective intelligence ensures that we arrive at the correct decision.

Feedback that might diminish the credibility of the resident in front of the patient should be reserved for an out-take discussion in the hallway.[12] Most commonly, this comes in the form of areas of improvement in interpersonal, communication, or professionalism skills. If the area for improvement was an action witnessed by the remainder of the team and the action was not egregious, it should be addressed in front of the remainder of the team. This ensures that the remainder of the team does not internalize the wrong action as appropriate. If it was an egregious action for which a reasonable person would clearly identify as unacceptable, a private conversation with the resident is most appropriate.

The moment after leaving the room is an opportunity for assessing and teaching residents' understanding of the severity of illness. In short, can residents identify which patients are "sick" versus "not sick?" The importance of the assessment can be established simply by asking, after each patient encounter, "What do you think? Is this patient sick or not sick?" The accuracy of the answer to each question is not as important as instilling the habit of asking the question, moving the subconscious impression of severity of illness into the consciousness.

Limitations and Reversals

Even with the best of strategy and tactics, there are situations whereby bedside rounds might not be the best approach. A patient with a mixed acid-base disorder, for example, might best be discussed via table-top rounds with a whiteboard, where complex diagrams and pictures can be drawn for instruction. Similarly, some patients might not feel comfortable being discussed in front of the entire team and there will be patients with complex family dynamics in the room; rounding individually with these patients might be the best course. It is also important to remember that the team has its physiologic needs, and occasional rounds at the table where food and beverages can be consumed can be useful.

It is important that patients are not excluded from bedside rounds merely because of physician convenience. Learning to overcome language barriers in delivering optimal health care is its own lesson, one to be mastered only by engaging in that care at the bedside. Excluding these patients from bedside rounds robs the team of mastering this skill and further perpetuates the attitude that underlies inequities of health care.

Giving bad news, apologizing for errors, and dealing with difficult patients are further examples whereby physician discomfort can lead to excluding these patients from bedside rounds. Learning how to overcome this discomfort becomes as much of a lesson as the conversation in question, and in each case is best learned by seeing the attending in action at the bedside.

SUMMARY

Though not suitable for every patient encounter, rounding at the beside provides an opportunity to teach and augment the attitudes essential for optimal medical care. It also provides an opportunity to establish and grow the team's culture as well as the culture for each patient encounter. Finally, it provides the attending with an opportunity to assess learners' position on the supervision-to-autonomy spectrum, thereby ensuring appropriate supervision while enabling the autonomy necessary for optimal learner growth.

DISCLOSURE

The authors have nothing to disclose.

REFERENCES

1. Gonzalo JD, Heist BS, Duffy BL, et al. The art of bedside rounds: a multi-center qualitative study of strategies used by experienced bedside teachers. J Gen Intern Med 2013;28:412–20.
2. Bloom BS, Engelhart MD, Furst EJ, et al. Taxonomy of educational objectives: the classification of educational goals. Handbook I: cognitive domain. New York: David McKay Company; 1956.
3. Lehmann LS, Brancati FL, Chen MC, et al. The effect of bedside case presentations on patients' perceptions of their medical care. N Engl J Med 1997;336: 1150–5.
4. Luthy C, Francis Gerstel P, Pugliesi A, et al. Bedside or not bedside: evaluation of patient satisfaction in intensive medical rehabilitation wards. PLoS One 2017;12: e0170474.
5. Ramirez J, Singh J, Williams AA. Patient satisfaction with bedside teaching rounds compared with nonbedside rounds. South Med J 2016;109:112–5.
6. Jacobowski NL, Girard TD, Mulder JA, et al. Communication in critical care: family rounds in the intensive care unit. Am J Crit Care 2010;19:421–30.
7. Chretien KC, Goldman EF, Craven KE, et al. A qualitative study of the meaning of physical examination teaching for patients. J Gen Intern Med 2010;25:786–91.
8. Gonzalo JD, Masters PA, Simons RJ, et al. Attending rounds and bedside case presentations: medical student and medicine resident experiences and attitudes. Teach Learn Med 2009;21:105–10.

9. Gonzalo JD, Chuang CH, Huang G, et al. The return of bedside rounds: an educational intervention. J Gen Intern Med 2010;25:792–8.

10. Gamp M, Becker C, Tondorf T, et al. Effect of bedside vs. non-bedside patient case presentation during ward rounds: a systematic review and meta-analysis. J Gen Intern Med 2019;34:447–57.

11. Gonzalo JD, Heist BS, Duffy BL, et al. The value of bedside rounds: a multicenter qualitative study. Teach Learn Med 2013;25:326–33.

12. Wiese JG. Teaching in the hospital. Philadelphia: American College of Physicians; 2010.

13. Noormohamadi SM, Arefi M, Afshaini K, et al. The effect of rational-emotive behavior therapy on anxiety and resilience in students. Int J Adolesc Med Health 2019. https://doi.org/10.1515/ijamh-2019-0099.

14. Harendza S, Krenz I, Klinge A, et al. Implementation of a Clinical Reasoning Course in the Internal Medicine trimester of the final year of undergraduate medical training and its effect on students' case presentation and differential diagnostic skills. GMS J Med Educ 2017;34(5):Doc66.

15. Cohen DL. Hand washing is all about respect for patients. BMJ Qual Saf 2016; 25(6):475.

16. Bruera E, Palmer JL, Pace E, et al. A randomized, controlled trial of physician postures when breaking bad news to cancer patients. Palliat Med 2007;21:501–5.

17. Merel SE, McKinney CM, Ufkes P, et al. Sitting at patients' bedsides may improve patients' perceptions of physician communication skills. J Hosp Med 2016;11: 865–8.

18. Swayden KJ, Anderson KK, Connelly LM, et al. Effect of sitting vs. standing on perception of provider time at bedside: a pilot study. Patient Educ Couns 2012; 86:166–71.

19. Johnson RL, Sadosty AT, Weaver AL, et al. To sit or not to sit? Ann Emerg Med 2008;51:188–93, 93.e1-2.

Moving?

Make sure your subscription moves with you!

To notify us of your new address, find your **Clinics Account Number** (located on your mailing label above your name), and contact customer service at:

Email: journalscustomerservice-usa@elsevier.com

800-654-2452 (subscribers in the U.S. & Canada)
314-447-8871 (subscribers outside of the U.S. & Canada)

Fax number: 314-447-8029

Elsevier Health Sciences Division
Subscription Customer Service
3251 Riverport Lane
Maryland Heights, MO 63043

*To ensure uninterrupted delivery of your subscription, please notify us at least 4 weeks in advance of move.

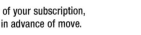

Printed and bound by CPI Group (UK) Ltd, Croydon, CR0 4YY

03/10/2024

01040407-0018